Pediatrics

Editor

AUTUMN P. DAVIDSON

VETERINARY CLINICS
OF NORTH AMERICA:
SMALL ANIMAL PRACTICE

www.vetsmall.theclinics.com

March 2014 • Volume 44 • Number 2

ELSEVIER

1600 John F. Kennedy Boulevard • Suite 1800 • Philadelphia, Pennsylvania, 19103-2899
http://www.vetsmall.theclinics.com

**VETERINARY CLINICS OF NORTH AMERICA: SMALL ANIMAL PRACTICE Volume 44, Number 2
March 2014 ISSN 0195-5616, ISBN-13: 978-0-323-28728-9**

Editor: Patrick Manley
Developmental Editor: Susan Showalter

Veterinary Clinics of North America: Small Animal Practice (ISSN 0195-5616) is published bimonthly by Elsevier Inc., 360 Park Avenue South, New York, NY 10010-1710. Months of issue are January, March, May, July, September, and November. Business and Editorial Offices: 1600 John F. Kennedy Blvd., Ste. 1800, Philadelphia, PA 19103-2899. Customer Service Office: 3251 Riverport Lane, Maryland Heights, MO 63043. Periodicals postage paid at New York, NY and additional mailing offices. Subscription prices are $310.00 per year (domestic individuals), $500.00 per year (domestic institutions), $150.00 per year (domestic students/residents), $410.00 per year (Canadian individuals), $621.00 per year (Canadian institutions), $455.00 per year (international individuals), $621.00 per year (international institutions), and $220.00 per year (international and Canadian students/residents). To receive student/resident rate, orders must be accompanied by name of affiliated institution, date of term, and the *signature* of program/residency coordinator on institution letterhead. Orders will be billed at individual rate until proof of status is received. Foreign air speed delivery is included in all *Clinics* subscription prices. All prices are subject to change without notice. **POSTMASTER:** Send address changes to *Veterinary Clinics of North America: Small Animal Practice*, Elsevier Health Sciences Division, Subscription Customer Service, 3251 Riverport Lane, Maryland Heights, MO 63043. Customer Service (orders, claims, online, change of address): Elsevier Periodicals Customer Service, Elsevier Health Sciences Division Subscription Customer Service 3251 Riverport Lane Maryland Heights, MO 63043. Tel: 1-800-654-2452 (U.S. and Canada); 314-447-8871 (outside U.S. and Canada). Fax: 314-447-8029. E-mail: journalscustomerservice-usa@elsevier.com (for print support); journalsonlinesupport-usa@elsevier.com (for online support).

Reprints. For copies of 100 or more of articles in this publication, please contact the Commercial Reprints Department, Elsevier Inc., 360 Park Avenue South, New York, NY 10010-1710. Tel.: 212-633-3874; Fax: 212-633-3820; E-mail: reprints@elsevier.com.

Veterinary Clinics of North America: Small Animal Practice is also published in Japanese by Inter Zoo Publishing Co., Ltd., Aoyama Crystal-Bldg 5F, 3-5-12 Kitaaoyama, Minato-ku, Tokyo 107-0061, Japan.

Veterinary Clinics of North America: Small Animal Practice is covered in *Current Contents/Agriculture, Biology and Environmental Sciences, Science Citation Index, ASCA, MEDLINE/PubMed (Index Medicus), Excerpta Medica,* and *BIOSIS.*

Printed and bound by CPI Group (UK) Ltd, Croydon, CR0 4YY

Contributors

EDITOR

AUTUMN P. DAVIDSON, DVM, MS
Diplomate, American College of Veterinary Internal Medicine; Veterinary Medical Teaching Hospital Small Animal Clinic, Department of Medicine and Epidemiology, School of Veterinary Medicine, University of California, Davis, California; Pet Care Veterinary Hospital, East Campus, Santa Rosa, California

AUTHORS

AUTUMN P. DAVIDSON, DVM, MS
Diplomate, American College of Veterinary Internal Medicine; Veterinary Medical Teaching Hospital Small Animal Clinic, Department of Medicine and Epidemiology, School of Veterinary Medicine, University of California, Davis, California; Pet Care Veterinary Hospital, East Campus, Santa Rosa, California

GINA M. DAVIS-WURZLER, DVM
Diplomate, American Board of Veterinary Practitioners, Canine and Feline Practice; Associate Health Sciences Clinical Professor, Outpatient Medicine, Department of Veterinary Medicine and Epidemiology, School of Veterinary Medicine, University of California-Davis; Service Chief, Small Animal Outpatient Medicine Service, William R. Pritchard Veterinary Medical Teaching Hospital, Davis, California

PATRICIA DEDRICK, DVM
Dedrick Veterinary Services, Santa Ynez, California

NADINE FIANI, BVSc
Diplomate, American Veterinary Dental College; Small Animal Specialist Hospital, Sydney, New South Wales, Australia

AMY J. FULTON, DVM
Dentistry and Oral Surgery Service, William R. Pritchard Veterinary Medical Teaching Hospital Small Animal Clinic, School of Veterinary Medicine, University of California-Davis, Davis; Cordova Veterinary Hospital, Rancho Cordova, California

DEBORAH S. GRECO, DVM, PhD
Diplomate, American College of Veterinary Internal Medicine; Nestle Purina PetCare, St Louis, Missouri

CLARE GREGORY, DVM
Diplomate, American College of Veterinary Surgery; Pet Care Veterinary Hospital, Santa Rosa, California

JAMES A. LAVELY, DVM
Diplomate, American College of Veterinary Internal Medicine–Neurology; Department of Neurology and Neurosurgery, VCA Animal Care Center of Sonoma, Rohnert Park, California

LISA PESCH, DVM With Thesis
Owner, Animal Healing Arts; Associate Veterinarian, Pet Care Veterinary Hospital, East
Campus, Holistic Medicine, Holistic Medicine; Adjunct Faculty, Veterinary Technology
Program, Agriculture & Natural Resources, Santa Rosa Junior College, Santa Rosa,
California

MARGARET V. ROOT KUSTRITZ, DVM, PhD
Diplomate of the American College of Theriogenologists; Department of Veterinary
Clinical Sciences, University of Minnesota College of Veterinary Medicine, St Paul,
Minnesota

JANE E. SYKES, BVSc(Hon), PhD
Diplomate, American College of Veterinary Internal Medicine; Professor, Department of
Medicine and Epidemiology, University of California-Davis, Davis, California

FRANK J.M. VERSTRAETE, DrMedVet, MMedVet
Diplomate, American Veterinary Dental College; Diplomate, European College of
Veterinary Surgeons; Diplomate, European Veterinary Dental College; Professor of
Dentistry and Oral Surgery, Department of Surgical and Radiological Sciences,
School of Veterinary Medicine, University of California-Davis, Davis, California

BENITA von DEHN, DVM
Diplomate of the American College of Veterinary Internal Medicine; Small Animal Internal
Medicine Consultant, Idexx Laboratories Inc, Westbrook, Maine; Department of Small
Animal Medicine, Pet Care Veterinary Hospital, East Campus, Santa Rosa, California

JODI L. WESTROPP, DVM, PhD
Diplomate of the American College of Veterinary Internal Medicine; Department of
Veterinary Medicine and Epidemiology, School of Veterinary Medicine, University of
California-Davis, Davis, California

Contents

Prudent veterinary intervention in the prenatal, parturient, and postpartum periods can increase neonatal survival by controlling or eliminating factors contributing to puppy morbidity and mortality. Postresuscitation or within the first 24 hours of a natural delivery, a complete physical examination should be performed by a veterinarian, technician, or knowledgeable breeder. Adequate ingestion of colostrum must occur promptly (within 24 hours) postpartum for puppies and kittens to acquire passive immunity.

This article provides clinically relevant and applicable information about normal biochemical values in puppies and kittens younger than 6 months, and is intended to provide practical guidelines for the interpretation of serum biochemical results in these young animals. At present there are no published sets of normal hematologic reference ranges for mixed-breed puppies and kittens younger than 6 months. Reference-value sets for closed research colonies composed of a few selected breeds are available, which help to provide insight into trends in normal hematologic and biochemical values for puppies and kittens.

Pediatric gonadectomy is most commonly performed by humane organizations as a means of population control. Benefits and detriments of gonadectomy are reviewed, with special attention to literature describing effects specific to age at gonadectomy. Techniques for pediatric anesthesia and surgery are reviewed.

Vaccines remain one of the practitioner's greatest tools in preventing disease and maintaining individual and population health. This article is an update to "Current Vaccination Strategies in Puppies and Kittens" published in *Veterinary Clinics of North America, Small Animal Practitioner*, in May 2006. There are now comprehensive guidelines readily available for small animal practitioners regarding canine and feline pediatric (and adult) vaccination recommendations. Perhaps more importantly, there is an increased dialogue regarding all aspects of preventive medicine, of which vaccination is only a small, yet significant portion; and an increased drive to provide scientific evidence for developing vaccination recommendations.

This article discusses pediatric nutrition in puppies and kittens. Supplementation of basic nutrients such as fat, protein, minerals, vitamins, and essential fatty acids of the bitch is essential for the proper growth and development of puppies during the lactation period. Milk replacers are compared for use in puppies and kittens. Supplements such as colostrum and probiotics for promotion of a healthy immune system and prevention or treatment of stress-induced and weaning diarrhea are also discussed.

Seizure disorders in young animals pose different considerations as to cause and therapeutic decisions compared with adult animals. Infectious diseases of the nervous system are more likely in puppies and kittens compared with adults. The diagnosis of canine distemper is often based on clinical signs. Idiopathic epilepsy typically occurs in dogs between 1 and 5 years of age; however, inflammatory brain diseases such as necrotizing encephalitis and granulomatous meningoencephalomyelitis also commonly occur in young to middle-aged small-breed dogs. The choice of which anticonvulsant to administer for maintenance therapy is tailored to each individual patient.

The oral examination is an important part of the physical examination of every patient. In neonate and adolescent dogs, it is important to inspect the oral cavity for congenital and acquired dental and oral pathology. This article reviews the more common pediatric and juvenile dental anomalies that affect dogs in order to provide a resource for the basic understanding of the oral cavity in these patients.

Congenital palate defects (CP) occur in dogs. Secondary cleft palate (SCP) is a congenital oronasal fistula resulting in incomplete closure of the hard and soft palate. SCP occurs alone or in combination with primary cleft palate involving the lip and premaxilla. CP results from incomplete fusion of the palatine shelves, most critical at 25 to 28 days gestation. Methods to improve survival of puppies with CP are sought by clients. This case report illustrates a successful method to manage nutrition in affected dogs until adult size is attained, facilitating surgical correction.

Infectious feline upper respiratory tract disease (URTD) continues to be a widespread and important cause of morbidity and mortality in kittens. Multiple pathogens can contribute to URTD in kittens, and coinfections are common in overcrowded environments and contribute to increased disease severity. Worldwide, the most prevalent pathogens are feline herpesvirus-1 and feline calicivirus. Primary bacterial causes of URTD in cats include *Bordetella bronchiseptica*, *Chlamydia felis*, and *Mycoplasma* species. *Streptococcus canis* and *Streptococcus equi* subspecies *zooepidemicus* occasionally play a role as primary pathogens in shelter situations and catteries. This article reviews the major causes of disease in kittens, and provides an update on treatment and prevention strategies.

 A video of laser revision of ectopic ureter accompanies this article

Ectopic ureters are the most common cause of urinary incontinence in young dogs but should be considered as a differential in any incontinent dog for which the history is not known. Ectopic ureters can be diagnosed with excretory urography, fluoroscopic urethrography or ureterography, abdominal ultrasonography, cystoscopy, helical computed tomography, or a combination of these diagnostic procedures. Other congenital abnormalities can also occur in dogs with ectopic ureters, including renal agenesis or dysplasia, hydronephrosis, and/or hydroureter and vestibulovaginal anomalies; therefore, the entire urinary system must be evaluated with ultrasonography if cystoscopy is the only other diagnostic tool used before surgery. Novel surgical techniques and adjunctive medical management have improved the prognosis for dogs with urinary ectopia.

Holistic veterinary medicine treats the whole patient including all physical and behavioral signs. The root cause of disease is treated at the same time as accompanying clinical signs. Herbal and nutritional supplements can help support tissue healing and proper organ functioning, thereby reducing the tendency of disease progression over time. Proper selection of homeopathic remedies is based on detailed evaluation of clinical signs. Herbal medicines are selected based on organ(s) affected and the physiologic nature of the imbalance. Many herbal and nutraceutical companies provide support for veterinarians, assisting with proper formula selection, dosing, drug interactions, and contraindications.

VETERINARY CLINICS OF NORTH AMERICA: SMALL ANIMAL PRACTICE

RELATED INTEREST

Veterinary Clinics of North America: Exotic Animal Practice
May 2012, Volume 15, Number 2
Pediatrics of Common and Uncommon Species
Kristine Kuchinski Broome, *Editor*

THE CLINICS ARE NOW AVAILABLE ONLINE!
Access your subscription at:
www.theclinics.com

Preface
Update: Small Animal Pediatrics

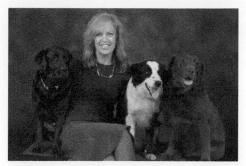

Autumn P. Davidson, DVM, MS, DACVIM
Editor

Pediatric patients continue to be the darlings of veterinary practice. They are, of course, endearing just in themselves. In my reproductive practice, the litter exam is often the rewarding end result and highlight of a challenging subfertility case. Pediatric patients offer the opportunity to begin the veterinarian:client:patient relationship anew when presented by their enthusiastic owner. The veterinarian has the perfect opportunity to educate about preventative medicine and dentistry, behavior modification, infectious and parasitic disease control, and neutering.

But veterinary pediatrics is challenging. Our patients are small and fragile; technology is limited, and resources are often restricted. Recognition of congenital and acquired disorders with a heritable basis requires diplomacy. Controversies fueled by the Internet now surround the very basics of veterinary pediatrics: vaccination and neutering.

Again, I heartily thank the busy veterinarians who took time from their clinical and academic practices to contribute to this update in veterinary pediatrics. As always, I learned a lot from reading their articles and I am proud to share them with our profession.

Autumn P. Davidson, DVM, MS, DACVIM
Veterinary Medical Teaching Hospital Small Animal Clinic
Department of Medicine and Epidemiology
School of Veterinary Medicine
University of California
1 Shields Avenue
Davis, CA 95616, USA

Pet Care Veterinary Hospital
East Campus, 2425 Mendocino Avenue
Santa Rosa, CA 95403, USA

E-mail address:
apdavidson@ucdavis.edu

Vet Clin Small Anim 44 (2014) ix
http://dx.doi.org/10.1016/j.cvsm.2013.12.001
0195-5616/14/$ – see front matter © 2014 Elsevier Inc. All rights reserved.

vetsmall.theclinics.com

Neonatal Resuscitation
Improving the Outcome

Autumn P. Davidson, DVM, MS

KEYWORDS

- Neonatal resuscitaion • Prenatal • Parturient • Postpartum

KEY POINTS

- Prudent veterinary intervention in the prenatal, parturient, and postpartum periods can increase neonatal survival by controlling or eliminating factors contributing to puppy morbidity and mortality.
- Postresuscitation or within the first 24 hours of a natural delivery, a complete physical examination should be performed by a veterinarian, technician, or knowledgeable breeder.
- Adequate ingestion of colostrum must occur promptly postpartum for puppies and kittens to acquire passive immunity.

The neonatal period can be defined as the first 2 weeks of postpartum life. Average reported neonatal mortality rates (greatest during the first week of life) vary, ranging from 9% to 26%. Prudent veterinary intervention in the prenatal, parturient, and postpartum periods can increase neonatal survival by controlling or eliminating factors contributing to puppy morbidity and mortality. Poor prepartum condition of the dam, dystocia, congenital malformations, genetic defects, injury, environmental exposure, malnutrition, parasitism, and infectious disease all contribute to neonatal morbidity and mortality. Optimal husbandry has an impact on neonatal survival favorably by managing labor and delivery to reduce stillbirths, controlling parasitism and reducing infectious disease, preventing injury and environmental exposure, and optimizing nutrition of the dam and neonates. Proper genetic screening for selection of breeders minimizes inherited congenital defects. The quality of labor (length, ease of the birth process, and quality of obstetric manipulation) has an impact on neonatal survival for up to 2 weeks postpartum. Proper neonatal resuscitation technique has a great impact on early neonatal survival. Neonatal resuscitation becomes necessary if the dam is anesthetized for a cesarean section, rejects the neonates or is ambivalent about immediate postpartum care, or is debilitated. Intervention for resuscitation of neonates after vaginal delivery should take place if a dam's actions fail to stimulate

Veterinary Medical Teaching Hospital Small Animal Clinic, Department of Medicine and Epidemiology, School of Veterinary Medicine, University of California, 1 Shields Avenue, Davis, CA 95616, USA; Pet Care Veterinary Hospital, East Campus, 2425 Mendocino Avenue, Santa Rosa, CA 95403, USA
E-mail address: apdavidson@ucdavis.edu

Vet Clin Small Anim 44 (2014) 191–204
http://dx.doi.org/10.1016/j.cvsm.2013.11.005
0195-5616/14/$ – see front matter © 2014 Elsevier Inc. All rights reserved.

vetsmall.theclinics.com

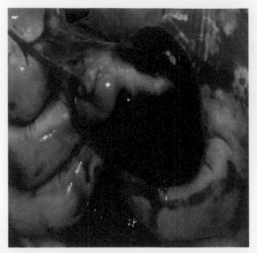

Fig. 1. Removal of fetal membranes from neonatal muzzle.

respiration, vocalization, and movement within 1 minute of birth. Increased veterinary participation in the resuscitation process can also be helpful if dystocia has contributed to poor postpartum condition of either the neonates or the dam.

Optimal neonatal resuscitation after birth (if the dam fails to do so) or cesarean section involves the same ABCs as any cardiopulmonary resuscitation. Spontaneous breathing and vocalization at birth are positively associated with survival through 7 days of age. Neonates delivered anesthetized via cesarean section often do not initiate respiration spontaneously. First, prompt clearing of airways (A = airway) by removing the fetal membranes from the face followed by gentle suction with a bulb syringe or aspirator should occur (**Figs. 1–3**). Removal of airway fluids is facilitated by lowering a neonate's head below the thorax (**Fig. 4**). Gentle but brisk drying and stimulation of the neonate with a small warm towel to promote respiration (B = breathing) and avoid chilling are performed (**Fig. 5**). Neonates should not be swung to clear airways as described in the veterinary and layman literature, because of the potential for cerebral hemorrhage from concussion. The use of doxapram as a respiratory stimulant is unlikely to improve hypoxemia associated with hypoventilation and is not recommended.

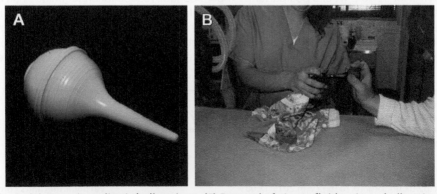

Fig. 2. (*A*) Preemie pediatric bulb syringe. (*B*) Removal of airway fluids using a bulb syringe.

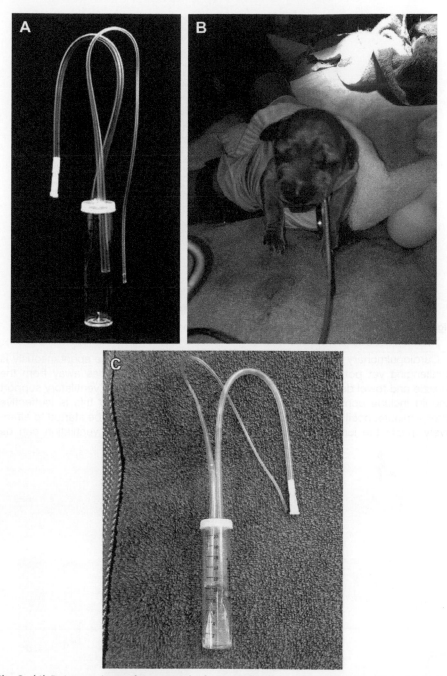

Fig. 3. (*A*) DeLee aspirator for removal of airway fluid. (*B*) DeLee aspirator placed in neonate's upper airway. (*C*) DeLee aspirator trap filled with airway fluid.

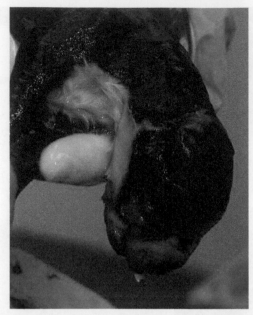

Fig. 4. Lowering the neonatal head facilitates fluid evacuation from the airways.

Cardiopulmonary resuscitation for neonates who fail to breathe spontaneously is challenging yet potentially rewarding. If clearing fetal membranes away from the muzzle and towel drying have not produced effective respiration, ventilatory support should include constant flow oxygen delivery by face mask. If this is ineffective after 1 minute, positive pressure with a snugly fitting mask should be started to effectively inflate the lungs (**Fig. 6**). Alternatively, positive pressure ventilation can be

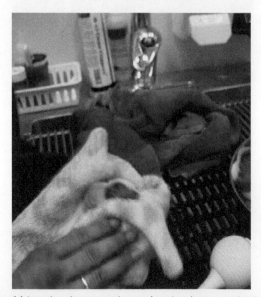

Fig. 5. Brisk gently rubbing the thorax and muzzle stimulates respiration.

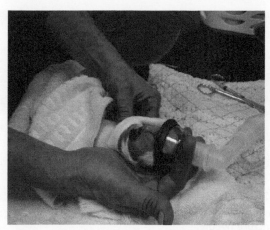

Fig. 6. Small, snugly fitting face mask permits oxygen flow by or positive pressure ventilation.

accomplished with a commercially available piglet resuscitator, which acts as an bag valve mask (**Fig. 7**). Endotracheal intubation and use of a rebreathing bag (using a 2-mm endotracheal tube or a 12- to 16-gauge intravenous catheter) is feasible but more technically difficult due to patient size and fragility and has more potential for trauma of the upper airway; 30 to 40 breaths per minute, with Fio_2 less than 40% to 60% and approximately 10 cm H_2O pressure, are advised. Effective ventilatory support causes the thorax to expand, indicating lung inflation. Excessive insufflation can cause aerophagia. Success at stimulating respiration with Jen Chung acupuncture point (GV 26) stimulation has been claimed when a small-gauge or acupuncture needle is inserted into the nasal philtrum at the base of the nares and rotated when cartilage/bone is contacted (**Fig. 8**). Drying the muzzle and Jen Chung likely stimulate respiratory neuroreceptors present in the muzzle and functional at birth.

Cardiac stimulation (C = circulation) should follow ventilatory support. Myocardial hypoxemia is the most common cause of bradycardia or asystole in the neonate.

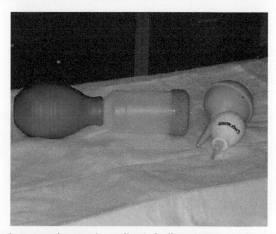

Fig. 7. Piglet resuscitator and preemie pediatric bulb syringes.

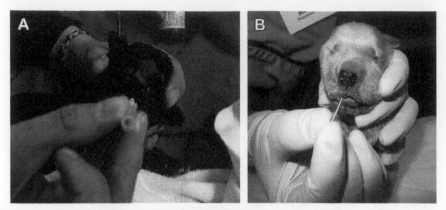

Fig. 8. Jen Chung acupressure point for stimulating respiration (*A*) Using a 25 G needle. (*B*) Using a 38 G acupuncture needle.

Improving oxygenation with positive pressure ventilation results in improved myocardial function; the neonatal heart rate improves. If bradycardia persists despite airway clearing and ventilation, direct transthoracic cardiac compressions are advised as the first step; epinephrine is the drug of choice for cardiac arrest/standstill (10–200 μg/kg or 0.01–0.20 μg/g) administered best by the intravenous or intraosseous route). Intratracheal dosage is not likely effective in the neonate and intracardiac puncture is traumatic. Epinephrine should be freshly diluted for neonatal resuscitation to permit accurate dosing. Venous access in the neonate is challenging; the single umbilical vein is one possibility if not already thrombosed; otherwise, a cephalic or the jugular vein can be accessed and eventually catheterized if intravenous fluids or therapy is desired (**Fig. 9**). The proximal humerus, proximal femur, and proximomedial tibia offer better, intraosseous sites for drug administration (**Fig. 10**). Circulation must be present for drug distribution; cardiac massage should continue after administration until a heartbeat is detectable. Atropine is currently not advised in neonatal resuscitation. The mechanism of bradycardia is hypoxemia-induced myocardial depression rather than vagal mediation, and anticholinergic-induced tachycardia can actually exacerbate myocardial oxygen deficits.

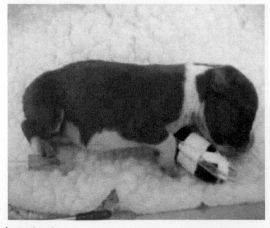

Fig. 9. Cephalic catheterization.

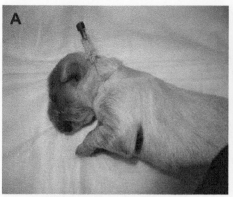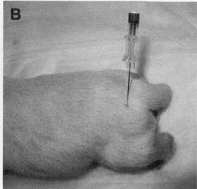

Fig. 10. Proximal (*A*) humeral and (*B*) femoral sites for intraosseous access.

BEYOND THE ABCS

When neonates fail to respond to routine resuscitation tactics, contributory factors should be considered. Chilled neonates can fail to respond to resuscitation. Loss of body temperature occurs rapidly when a neonate is damp. Keeping neonates warm is important during resuscitation and in the immediate postpartum period. During resuscitation, placing a chilled neonate's body into a warm water bath (95°F–99°F) can improve core temperature (**Fig. 11**). Thoracic compressions and oxygenation by face mask can continue while a neonate is in the water bath. Working under a heat lamp or a Bair hugger warming device is helpful in managing chilling during resuscitation. Postresuscitation, neonates should be placed in a warm box (a Styrofoam picnic box with ventilation holes is ideal) with warm bedding until they can be safely left with their dam (**Fig. 12**).

Hypoglycemia also results in a poor response to resuscitation. Neonates lack glucose reserves and have minimal capacity for gluconeogenesis. Providing energy during prolonged resuscitation efforts becomes critical. Clinical hypoglycemia involves blood glucose levels less than 30 to 40 mg/dL and can be treated with dextrose solution, given either intravenously/intraosseously, at a dose of 0.5 to

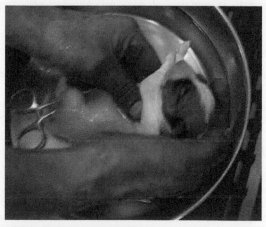

Fig. 11. Warm water bath during resuscitation.

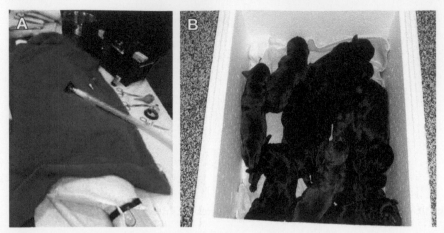

Fig. 12. (*A*) Bair hugger supplies a warm surface for resuscitation. Resuscitation equipment is tableside. (*B*) Simple but effective postresuscitation housing in a Styrofoam box with heat support.

1.0 g/kg body weight (0.0005–0.001 g/gram body weight) using a 5% to 10% dextrose solution, or at a dose of 2 to 4 mL/kg body weight (0.002–0.004 mL/gram body weight) of a 10% dextrose solution. Venous access is challenging in tiny neonates. Subcutaneous administration is undesirable due to the potential for abscessation at the site. A single administration of parenteral glucose is adequate if a puppy then nurses or can be fed; 50% dextrose solution should only be applied to the mucous membranes because of the potential for phlebitis if administered intravenously; however, circulation must be adequate for absorption from the mucosa or gastrointestinal tract, and there is a risk of aspiration. Neonates administered multiple doses of dextrose should be monitored for hyperglycemia because of immature metabolic regulatory mechanisms. If a neonate is too weak to nurse or suckle, a mixture of a warmed, balanced half-strength saline with 2.5% dextrose (so as not to be hypertonic) may be administered by stomach tube at a dose of 0.1 to 0.5 mL per 30 g of body weight, until the puppy can be fed or nurses. A balanced warmed dextrose-electrolyte solution can be administered orally by stomach tube every 15 to 30 minutes until the neonate is capable of suckling. Alternatively, acquiring colostrum from the dam is superior for this purpose.

WHEN TO STOP RESUSCITATION

1. No response after 15 to 20 minutes of effort (continued agonal respiration or bradycardia)
2. Serious congenital defect detected (cleft palate, loud murmur, gastroschisis, large omphalocele, large fontanel, anasarca, or anogenital defect) (**Figs. 13–15**)

UMBILICAL CORD MANAGEMENT

Umbilical cord care should take place after the neonate is resuscitated (is vocal, moving, and pink). The umbilicus of neonates should be treated with 2% tincture of iodine immediately after birth to reduce contamination and prevent ascent of bacteria into the peritoneal cavity (omphalitis-peritonitis). Alcohol-based tincture of iodine is superior to betadyne, which is water based and does not promote umbilical desiccation as

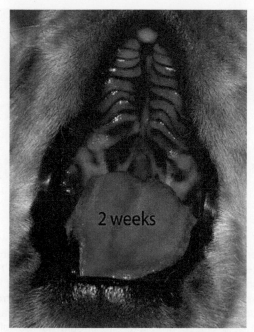

Fig. 13. Complete soft and hard palate cleft.

quickly. After cutting the cord with clean scissors approximately 0.5 to 1.0 cm from the abdominal wall, or trimming it if the dam removed the placenta and nipped the cord, the cord should be ligated with suture and dunked thoroughly in 2% iodine (**Fig. 16**).

HUSBANDRY: THE FIRST DAYS

Postresuscitation or within the first 24 hours of a natural delivery, a complete physical examination should be performed by a veterinarian, technician, or knowledgeable breeder. Neonates should be individually identified if similar in appearance to facilitate record keeping using clipping (small patch on right or left shoulder, right or left hip, tail base, or top of head) or dot of nail polish. The use of small collars is less desirable due

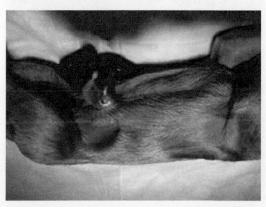

Fig. 14. Omphalocele.

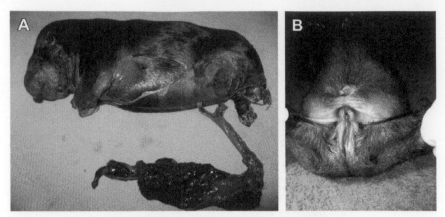

Fig. 15. (*A*) Anasarca. (*B*) Anogenital defect.

to the potential for entrapment of limbs and choking. The oral cavity, hair coat, limbs, umbilicus, and urogenital structures should be visually inspected. The mucous membranes should be pink and moist, a suckle reflex present, the coat full and clean, and the urethra and anus patent. A normal umbilicus is dry without surrounding erythema (**Fig. 17**). An umbilical hernia is of concern if large enough to entrap bowel. Omental entrapment outside of a closed umbilical site should not be misinterpreted as a body wall defect. No urine should be evident at the umbilicus (patent urachus). The thorax should be auscultated; vesicular breath sounds and a lack of murmur are normal. The abdomen should be pliant and not painful. A normal neonate squirms and vocalizes when examined and nurses and sleeps quietly when returned to the dam and litter. Normal neonates attempt to right themselves and orient by rooting toward their dam using the olfactory and tactile senses. Neonates are highly susceptible to environmental stress, infection, and malnutrition. Proper husbandry is critical and should include daily examination of each neonate for vigor and recording of weight. Lack of weight gain or actual weight loss is the first signs in a neonate failing to thrive. Postresuscitation, each neonate should be weighed and recorded for the owner to follow-up with daily (**Fig. 18**).

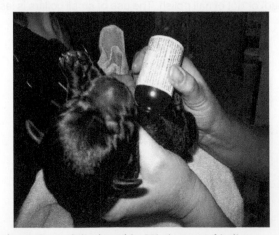

Fig. 16. Dunking the entire umbilical cord in 2% tincture of iodine.

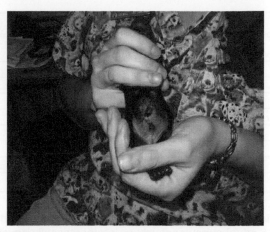

Fig. 17. Normal appearance of ligated umbilicus.

WARMTH

Neonates lack thermoregulatory mechanisms until 4 weeks of age; thus, the ambient temperature must be high enough to facilitate maintenance of a body temperature of at least 97°F (36°C) **(Table 1)**. Hypothermia has a negative impact on immunity, nursing, and digestion. Exogenous heat should be supplied, best in the form of an overhead heat lamp. Heating pads run the risk of burning neonates incapable of moving away from excessively hot surfaces.

Postresuscitation, chilled older neonates must be rewarmed slowly (30 minutes) to avoid peripheral vasodilation and dehydration. Tube feeding should be delayed until the neonate is euthermic; hypothermia induces ileus and regurgitation and aspiration can result.

IMMUNITY

Incompletely developed immune systems during the first 10 days of life make neonates vulnerable to systemic infection (most commonly bacterial and viral). Adequate ingestion of colostrum must occur promptly postpartum for puppies and kittens to acquire passive immunity. The intestinal absorption of IgG generally ceases by

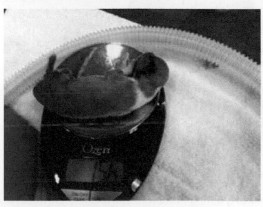

Fig. 18. Gram scale for neonatal weighing.

Table 1
Normal body temperatures and environmental warmth required for neonates

Neonatal normal body temperature (rectal)	
Week 1	95°F–99°F
Week 2–3	97°F–100°F
At weaning	99°F–101°F
Environmental warmth required	
Week 1	84°F–89°F
Week 2/3	80°F
Week 4	69°F–75°F
Week 5	69°F

24 hours after parturition. Colostrum-deprived kittens given adult cat serum at a dose of 150 mL/kg (0.15 mL/g) subcutaneously or intraperitoneally developed serum IgG levels comparable with suckling littermates; however, colostrum-deprived puppies given 40 mL/kg adult dog serum orally and parentally failed to match suckling littermates' IgG levels. Puppies likely require as much as 0.10 mL/g). The dose should be divided over several administrations. Colostrum or serum replacement can be given orally during the first 24 hours of life; thereafter, it must be given parenterally and intestinal absorption of macromolecules is compromised. The subcutaneous route is preferred to intraperitoneal administration. Neonates should be encouraged to suckle promptly after resuscitation is completed; this usually necessitates close monitoring after a cesarean section because the dam is still groggy from anesthesia (**Fig. 19**). Maternal instincts (protecting, retrieving, grooming, and nursing) usually return within 24 hours postanesthesia. The use of appropriate analgesics (narcotics) hastens good maternal behavior.

Neonatal bacterial septicemia can cause rapid deterioration, resulting in death if not recognized and treated promptly. Factors that reportedly predispose a puppy to septicemia include endometritis in the bitch, a prolonged delivery/dystocia, feeding of replacement formulas, the use of ampicillin, stress, low birth weight (<350 g for a medium-sized breed), and chilling with body temperature less than 96°. The organisms most frequently associated with septicemia are *Escherichia coli*, *Streptococci*,

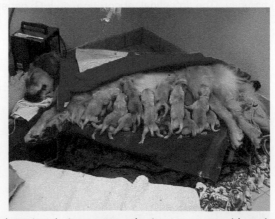

Fig. 19. Supervised nursing during postanesthesia recovery provides valuable glucose, calories, and immunoglobulins to neonates.

Staphylococci, and *Klebsiella* spp. Premortem diagnosis can be challenging; clinical signs may not be noted due to sudden death. Commonly, a decrease in weight gain, failure to suckle, hematuria, persistent diarrhea, unusual vocalization, abdominal distension and pain, and sloughing of the extremities indicate septicemia may be present. Prompt therapy with broad-spectrum, bactericidal antibiotics, and improved nutrition via supported nursing, tube feeding or bottle-feeding, maintenance of body temperature, and appropriate fluid replacement are indicated. The third-generation cephalosporin antibiotic ceftiofur sodium (Naxcel, Pharmacia & Upjohn, Kalamazoo, Michigan) is an appropriate choice for neonatal septicemia because it alters normal intestinal flora minimally and is usually effective against the causative organisms. Ceftiofur sodium should be administered at a dose of 2.5 mg/kg (0.0025 mg/g) subcutaneously every 12 hours for no longer than 5 days. Because puppies less than 48 hours old have reduced thrombin levels, presumptive therapy with vitamin K_1 may be used (0.01–1.0 mg subcutaneously per puppy) (**Box 1**, **Fig. 20**).

GROCERIES

Neonates have minimal body fat reserves and limited metabolic capacity to generate glucose from precursors. Glycogen stores are depleted shortly after birth, making

---

Box 1
Contents of neonatal resuscitation kit

Neonatal Resuscitation Kit

- Tuberculin syringe (TB), acupuncture needles, very small gauge needles ≤25 G
- Epinephrine freshly diluted 1:9, 50% dextrose freshly diluted to 5%
- Oxygen sources
- Suction (pediatric bulb syringes)
- DeLee aspirators
- Small face masks
- Towels (small)
- Heat source (Bair hugger, warm water blanket, infrared lamp)
- Puppy box (Styrofoam) with heat support
- Multiple clean mosquito forceps and small scissors
- 3-0 Gut suture for umbilical cords needle removed, cut in 5″ lengths
- Tincture of iodine 2%
- Bowls for warm water baths
- Pediatric/neonatal stethoscope
- Doppler
- Neonatal scale

Neonatal Resuscitation Drugs

- Dilute epinephrine
- Dilute dextrose
- Ceftiofur reconstitute, dilute and freeze for improved shelf life
- Vitamin K_1

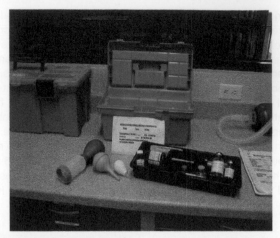

Fig. 20. Dedicated neonatal resuscitation kit.

adequate nourishment from nursing vital. Even minimal fasting can result in hypoglycemia. Hypoglycemia can also result from endotoxemia, septicemia, portosystemic shunts, and glycogen storage abnormalities. Oral fluid and glucose replacement may be preferable if a puppy has an adequate swallowing reflex and is not clinically compromised. The neonatal caloric requirement is 133 cal/kg/d during the first week of life, 155 cal/kg/d for the second, 175 to 198 cal/kg/d for the third, and 220 cal/kg/d for the fourth. Commercially manufactured milk replacement formulas (Esbilac and KMR, PetAg, Hampshire, Illinois; Eukanuba Puppy Milk Replacer Formula, Iams, Dayton, Ohio; and Veta-Lac, Lloyd, Shenandoah, Iowa) are usually superior to homemade versions. The use of milk obtained from the dam can be considered if available. An osmotic diarrhea (usually yellow, curdled stool appearance) can result from overfeeding formula, necessitating diluting the product 50% with water or a balanced crystalloid, such as lactated Ringer solution. Neonates should gain weight steadily from the first day after birth (a transient mild loss from birth weight is acceptable on day 1); puppies should gain 1 to 3 g per day per pound (2.2 kg) of anticipated adult weight and kittens 50 to 100 g weekly. Minimal weight gain of 10%/d should occur. Neonatal weights should be recorded daily for the first 2 weeks, then every 3 days until a month of age. Healthy, well-nourished neonates are quiet and sleep when not nursing.

FURTHER READINGS

Davidson A. Canine herpesvirus infection. In: Sykes J, editor. Canine and feline infectious diseases. St Louis (MO): Elsevier; 2013. p. 166–70.

Davidson A. The practice of theriogenology. In: Nelson R, Couto G, editors. Small animal internal medicine. St Louis (MO): Elsevier; 2013. p. 897–914.

Johnson C, Casal M. Neonatal resuscitation: canine and feline. In: Lopate C, editor. Management of pregnant and neonatal dogs, cats and exotic pets. Ames (IO): Wiley-Blackwell; 2012. p. 677–92.

Rickard V. Birth and the first 24 hours. In: Peterson M, Kutzler M, editors. Small animal pediatrics: the first 12 months of life. St Louis (MO): Elsevier-Saunders; 2011. p. 11–9.

Pediatric Clinical Pathology

Benita von Dehn, DVM

KEYWORDS

- Neonatal clinical pathology • Pediatric hematology • Urinary system
- Hepatobiliary system

KEY POINTS

- Because of variations in enzymology and functional capacity of neonatal organ systems, care must be taken when interpreting any changes in clinical chemistry values when using standard adult reference ranges.
- Although published reference ranges are provided, based on the available research in current literature it is recommended that these ranges are used only as guidelines, owing to the lack of standardization of reference intervals among reference laboratories.
- This article is not intended to provide a fully comprehensive review of all hematologic and biochemical changes that occur from birth to 6 months of age, but to help provide a practical guideline for interpretation and useful diagnostic information in determining the state of health or cause of illness in a young dog or cat.

INTRODUCTION

Neonates possess a decreased functional capacity of many organ systems and variations in enzyme levels, which improve in accordance with appropriate growth. Because of these physiologic developmental changes, care must be taken when interpreting any changes in clinical chemistry values when using standard adult reference ranges.

This article is intended to provide pertinent and applicable information about normal biochemical values in puppies and kittens younger than 6 months. The article is not intended to be a comprehensive review of small animal biochemistry and physiology, but rather aims to help provide practical guidelines for interpretation of serum biochemical results in puppies and kittens younger than 6 months.

At present there are no published sets of normal hematologic reference ranges for mixed-breed puppies and kittens younger than 6 months. Reference-value sets for closed research colonies composed of a few selected breeds are available, which help provide insight into trends in normal hematologic and biochemical values for puppies and kittens.

Idexx Laboratories Inc, 1 IDEXX Drive, Westbrook, Maine; Department of Small Animal Medicine, Pet Care Veterinary Hospital, East Campus, 2425 Mendocino Avenue, Santa Rosa, CA 95403, USA
E-mail address: docbenita@aol.com

Vet Clin Small Anim 44 (2014) 205–219
http://dx.doi.org/10.1016/j.cvsm.2013.10.003
0195-5616/14/$ – see front matter © 2014 Elsevier Inc. All rights reserved.

HEMATOPOIETIC SYSTEM

Normal physiologic changes reflected in the complete blood count results include a decline in hematocrit in the first several weeks of life. The hematocrit of the neonate may be high at birth, but declines dramatically by 3 days of age, and continues to decrease to adult normal range by 2 to 6 months of age.[1–4] The decreased production and shortened life span of the red blood cells (RBCs) can result in increased polychromasia, nucleated RBCs, Howell-Jolly bodies, and Heinz bodies (kittens only).[5,6] The neonate RBC exhibits macrocytosis, with mean corpuscular volume decreasing to that of adults by 4 weeks of age as fetal RBCs are replaced by adult RBCs.[7] Gradual progressive climb in hematologic parameters can be detected by 2 months of age, with adult reference ranges for RBC, hemoglobin, and hematocrit usually reached by 6 months. The guidelines for evaluating a regenerative response in adult animals is likely sufficient for puppies and kittens older than 4 months (**Tables 1** and **2**). A greater regenerative response should be observed in animals younger than 4 months.[2]

White blood cell (WBC) differential analysis for puppies and kittens younger than 6 months remains within the reference interval for adult animals. For puppies, the WBC count as well as neutrophil and lymphocyte counts are relatively high at birth, decline during the first month of life, increase by the second month, and then slowly decline. For kittens, WBC as well as neutrophil and lymphocyte counts at birth are well within the adult reference range, but increase to above the adult reference range for kittens at 3 to 4 months of age, then values return to within normal adult reference ranges by about 5 to 6 months of age.[1,2] This leukocytosis, usually comprising neutrophilia and lymphocytosis, may be a physiologic response resulting from excitement and immune stimulation (**Tables 1** and **3**).

Clinical Implications

Determining the cause of an anemia in a puppy or kitten is important, and may be vital in determining a diagnosis and subsequent treatment plan. Classifying the anemia into a pathophysiologic category of regenerative, iron-deficiency, or nonregenerative based on changes in the erythrogram may be useful. Elevated reticulocytes are the preferred method for evaluation of the regenerative response in puppies and kittens. Animals younger than 4 months should have a greater reticulocyte response than that considered to be regenerative in adult dogs and cats.[2] Once the anemia has been determined to be regenerative, the total plasma or serum protein concentration can be assessed to help determine if the cause of the anemia is hemolysis or hemorrhage. The total plasma protein concentration is usually low with hemorrhage. The common causes of blood-loss anemia in puppies and kittens include inherited or acquired coagulopathies, excessive hemorrhage after trauma or surgeries, and hematophagous parasitism. The hallmark of chronic blood loss and, ultimately, iron-deficiency anemia are microcytic hypochromic RBCs (low mean corpuscular volume and low mean corpuscular hemoglobin concentration).

By contrast, regenerative hemolytic anemias tend to demonstrate normal or increased serum (or plasma) total protein. Common causes of hemolytic anemias in puppies and kittens include immune-mediated hemolytic anemia, most often attributable to neonatal isoerythrolysis, oxidative injury, and Heinz body formation (ie, a variety of foods such as onions, garlic powder, certain drugs, and plant substances); microangiopathy (ie, feline infectious peritonitis); and hemoparasites (ie, hemotropic *Mycoplasma*, *Babesia*, cytauxzoonosis).

Nonregenerative anemias are uncommon in puppies and kittens, and are usually associated with underlying illnesses such as renal failure, endocrinopathies, and inflammatory, viral, or neoplastic diseases. A nonregenerative anemia may or may not be seen before 6 months of age with some chronic congenital disorders.

URINARY SYSTEM

Blood urea nitrogen (BUN) and creatinine are the most commonly assessed indices of glomerular filtration. Significant variability in the rate of maturation of intrinsic renal mechanisms regulating glomerular filtration rate (GFR), renal blood flow (RBF), and distal delivery of water and solute are observed in puppies and between species. GFR increases 7-fold over the first month of life in canine neonates. Similarly, RBF increases nearly 4-fold during the same period. Both GFR and RBF continue to increase after 4 weeks of age, reaching adult values approximately 10 weeks after birth. Studies in cats suggest that GFR in kittens also increases rapidly after birth, reaching adult values by 9 weeks of age.[11]

In the dog, the neonatal kidney is morphologically and functionally immature, with nephrogenesis continuing for at least 2 weeks after birth.[7] Newborn puppies possess a limited ability to concentrate or dilute urine in response to changes in extracellular fluid volume. Only limited information regarding nephrogenesis in the cat is available, and one must be cautious not to compare directly or make assumptions. The BUN level has consistently been shown to be lower in young animals when compared with adults. Of note, BUN is initially high (within adult values), then decreases between the ages of 2 weeks and 3 months, before beginning to increase again to obtain adult values by approximately 6 months of age. Proposed reasons for the lower BUN in puppies have been attributed to increased protein synthesis as a result of growth hormone influence or, possibly, increased metabolic state with increased GFR.[12] BUN is also initially high in kittens at birth and then decreases to below adult values in kittens younger than 8 weeks. Adult values are reached shortly thereafter.[12]

In neonatal puppies between 1 and 3 days of age, creatinine levels are high, with wide variation. A gradual progressive decrease occurs until 28 to 33 days of age followed by a slight increase at 7 to 8 weeks of age. Creatinine levels may then increase moderately up to 1 year of age. Breed variations in creatinine have been observed. German Shepherd puppies up to 8 weeks of age have reportedly higher creatinine values, and adult Greyhounds have higher creatinine concentrations because of their increased muscle mass.[12] In kittens, creatinine levels are also similarly high at birth, and then decrease to equivalent or less than adult levels through 8 weeks of age. Exactly when adult levels are actually reached in cats has not been reported. No breed variations have been reported in cats (See **Tables 4–7**).[12]

Autoregulation of RBF and GFR in neonatal puppies appears to be relatively inefficient in response to rapid changes in systemic arterial blood pressure. At birth, arterial pressure is low (50–60 mm Hg); during renal maturation, increased blood pressure and decreased vascular resistance result in an increase in GFR and RBF.[7] In the adult dog, the renin-angiotensin system is an important regulatory mechanism; however, in the neonate RBF is directly correlated with arterial pressure and does not seem to be altered by inhibition of the angiotensin until approximately 6 weeks of age.[7]

Maintenance of electrolyte balance is tightly regulated by the body, and occurs predominantly via renal tubular resorption and secretion of these electrolytes in response to hydration status, serum osmolality, and acid-base balance. Sodium balance appears to be relatively stable in newborn puppies. Whole kidney fractional resorption of sodium was constant in 2- to 77-day-old puppies and was similar to values in adult dogs. Nevertheless, puppies younger than 3 weeks appear to have impaired ability to

Table 1
Hematologic values for growing, healthy beagle dogs

Hematologic Parameter	Birth[a]	1[a]	2[a]	3[a]	4[a]	6[a]	8	Age (wk) 12[b]	16[b]	20[b]	24[b]	28[b]	40[b]	44[b]	52[b]
RBC (×10^6/µL)	4.7–5.6 (5.1)	3.6–5.9 (4.6)	3.4–4.4 (3.9)	3.5–4.3 (3.8)	3.6–4.9 (4.1)	4.3–5.1 (4.7)	4.5–5.9 (4.9)	(6.34)	(6.38)	(6.93)	(7.41)	(8.45)	(8.69)	(8.47)	(7.68)
Hemoglobin (g/dL)	14.0–17.0 (15.2)	10.4–17.5 (12.9)	9.0–11.0 (10.0)	8.6–11.6 (9.7)	8.5–10.3 (9.5)	8.5–11.3 (10.2)	10.3–12.5 (11.2)	14.3	15.0	16.0	16.7	17.7	18.2	18.8	18.1
PCV (%)	45.0–52.5 (47.5)	33.0–52.0 (40.5)	29.0–34.0 (31.8)	27.0–37.0 (31.7)	27.0–33.5 (29.9)	26.5–35.5 (32.5)	31.0–39.0 (34.8)	(40.9)	(43.0)	(44.9)	(47.6)	(48.8)	(50.8)	(50.2)	(49.3)
MCV (fL)	(93.0)	(89.0)	(81.5)	(83.0)	(73.0)	(69.0)	(72.0)	(64.6)	(67.4)	(64.8)	(64.2)	(57.8)	(58.4)	(59.3)	(63.5)
MCH (pg)	(30.0)	(28.0)	(25.5)	(25.0)	(23.0)	(22.0)	(22.5)	(22.8)	(23.5)	(23.0)	(22.5)	(20.5)	(20.9)	(22.1)	(23.6)
MCHC (%)	(32.0)	(32.0)	(31.5)	(31.0)	(32.0)	(31.5)	(32.0)	(35.3)	(34.8)	(35.6)	(35.1)	(36.1)	(35.9)	(37.3)	(37.1)
nRBC/100 WBC	0–13 (2.3)	0–11 (4.0)	0–6 (2.0)	0–9 (1.6)	0–4 (1.2)	0	0–1 (0.2)	—	—	—	—	—	—	—	—
Reticulocytes (%)	4.5–9.2 (6.5)	3.8–15.2 (6.9)	4.0–8.4 (6.7)	5.0–9.0 (6.9)	4.6–6.6 (5.8)	2.6–6.2 (4.5)	1.0–6.0 (3.6)	—	—	—	—	—	—	—	—
Total WBC (×10^3/µL)	6.8–18.4 (12.0)	9.0–23.0 (14.1)	8.1–15.1 (11.7)	6.7–15.1 (11.2)	8.5–16.4 (12.9)	12.6–26.7 (16.3)	12.7–17.3 (15.0)	17.1	16.3	14.6	15.6	15.5	14.4	13.9	14.0

Segmented neutrophils	4.4–15.8 (8.6)	3.8–15.2 (7.4)	3.2–10.4 (5.2)	1.4–9.4 (5.1)	3.7–12.8 (7.2)	4.2–17.6 (9.0)	6.2–11.8 (8.5)	(9.8)	(9.0)	(8.9)	(9.1)	(9.1)	(8.7)	(8.1)
Band neutrophils	0–1.5 (0.23)	0–4.8 (0.50)	0–1.2 (0.21)	0–0.5 (0.09)	0–0.3 (0.06)	0–0.3 (0.05)	0–0.3 (0.08)	(0.08)	(0.1)	(0.02)	(0.08)	(0.02)	(0.02)	(0.04)
Lymphocytes	0.5–4.2 (1.9)	1.3–9.4 (4.3)	1.5–7.4 (3.8)	2.1–10.1 (5.0)	1.0–8.4 (4.5)	2.8–16.6 (5.7)	3.1–6.9 (5.0)	(5.7)	(5.9)	(4.5)	(5.3)	(4.8)	(3.4)	(4.7)
Monocytes	0.2–2.2 (0.9)	0.3–2.5 (1.1)	0.2–1.4 (0.7)	0.1–1.4 (0.7)	0.3–1.5 (0.8)	0.5–2.7 (1.1)	0.4–1.7 (1.0)	(0.9)	(0.9)	(0.8)	(0.7)	(0.7)	(0.6)	(0.5)
Eosinophils	0–1.3 (0.4)	0.2–2.8 (0.8)	0.08–1.8 (0.6)	0.07–0.9 (0.3)	0–0.7 (0.25)	0.1–1.9 (0.5)	0–1.2 (0.4)	(0.4)	(0.4)	(0.3)	(0.5)	(0.8)	(0.5)	(0.5)
Basophils	—	0–0.2 (0.01)	—	—	0–0.15 (0.01)	—	—	—	—	—	—	—	—	—
Platelets (×10³/μL)	178–465 (302)	282–560 (352)	210–352 (290)	203–370 (272)	130–360 (287)	275–570 (371)	240–435 (324)	—	—	—	—	—	—	—

Values in parentheses are mean values.

Abbreviations: MCH, mean corpuscular hemoglobin; MCHC, mean corpuscular hemoglobin concentration; MCV, mean corpuscular volume; nRBC/100 WBC, number of nucleated red blood cells per 100 white blood cells; PCV, packed cell volume; RBC, red blood cells; total WBC, total white blood cell count.

a Normal ranges and/or mean values from Earl FL, Melveger BA, Wilson RL. The hemogram and bone marrow profile of normal neonatal and weanling beagle dogs. Lab Anim Sci 1973;23:690–5.

b Mean values from Anderson AC, Gee W. Normal blood values in the beagle. Vet Med 1958;53:135–8, 156.

Table 2
Regenerative response in puppies and kittens

PCV (%)	Puppies		Kittens	
	Polychromasia	Reticulocytes[a]	Polychromasia	Reticulocytes[a]
>25	1–2+	>80,000/μL	1–2+	>60,000/μL
15–25	2–3+	—	2–3+	—
<15	4+	—	4+	—

[a] These values represent the minimum absolute numbers of reticulocytes required for an interpretation of a regenerative response. If the packed cell volume (PCV) is lower, the absolute number of reticulocytes should increase proportionately.

excrete excess sodium in comparison with adult dogs.[11] In puppies, serum sodium and chloride concentrations are slightly lower at or before 6 weeks of age relative to adult levels. Serum potassium is low at age 2 to 4 weeks and then peaks at age 6 to 8 weeks, before gradually dropping off to values comparable with adult levels. This low serum potassium is presumed to be caused by the presence of sodium/potassium (Na/K) pumps in neonatal erythrocytes, resulting in higher concentrations of intracellular potassium (relative to extracellular concentrations) than exist in adult dogs. These Na/K pumps appear to be lost quickly after birth in most breeds of dogs, with the exception of Akitas, Jindos, and Japanese Shibas. Thus, these latter breeds of dogs have higher concentrations of intracellular potassium than other dog breeds.[12]

Age-associated differences have been noted for potassium and chloride in kittens; however, no differences have been found for sodium. Potassium is slightly lower in kittens younger than 3 months in comparison with older kittens. These values increase slightly between 4 and 6 months of age and then gradually decrease again to reach adult levels by 6 months. Chloride is lowest in kittens younger than 3 months, then increase to adult parameters by approximately 4 to 6 months of age.[12]

Significant differences in acid-base balance exist between puppies/kittens and adults. Neonatal puppies, but not kittens, have an impaired ability to increase renal ammoniagenesis in response to an acid environment when compared with adults. By 3 weeks of age, most amino acids are resorbed in puppies, and by 7 weeks of age adult patterns of amino acid resorption are evident. Incomplete tubular resorption of glucose is commonly observed in puppies (which may be related to a greater proportion of immature nephrons). Glucosuria was detected in 50% of urinalyses obtained from 5-day-old puppies, but was not detected in puppies aged 21 days or older.[11]

Clinical Implications

The immaturity of glomerular and renal tubular function has significant clinical implications with regard to therapeutic management of puppies and kittens. Puppies and kittens are predisposed to rapid dehydration as a result of their higher water requirements, and their decreased ability to concentrate urine and resist osmotic diuresis.[13] On the other hand, they are also more susceptible to fluid volume and solute overload. Judicious fluid administration and close monitoring is essential in managing immature animals. Recommended daily fluid rates for the canine neonate range from 60 to 180 mL/kg/d.[7]

Urine is relatively easily to obtain from the neonate with genital stimulation. As previously discussed, the immaturity of the neonatal kidney alters interpretation of the

Table 3
Hematologic values for growing, healthy cats

Hematologic Parameter	Age (wk)										
	0–2[a]	2–4[a]	4–6[a]	6–8[a]	8–9[a]	12–13[a]	16–17[a]	20[b]	30[b]	44[b]	52[b]
RBC (×10⁶/µL)	5.29 ± 0.24	4.67 ± 0.10	5.89 ± 0.23	6.57 ± 0.26	6.95 ± 0.09	7.43 ± 0.23	8.14 ± 0.27	7.4 ± 0.7	8.0 ± 0.5	7.9 ± 0.8	7.7 ± 0.8
Hemoglobin (g/dL)	12.1 ± 0.6	8.7 ± 0.2	8.6 ± 0.3	9.1 ± 0.3	9.8 ± 0.2	10.1 ± 0.3	11.0 ± 0.4	10.7 ± 1.2	12.1 ± 1.8	13.0 ± 2.1	13.3 ± 1.8
PCV (%)	35.3 ± 1.7	26.5 ± 0.8	27.1 ± 0.8	29.8 ± 1.3	33.3 ± 0.7	33.1 ± 1.6	34.9 ± 1.1	33.4 ± 3.3	37.1 ± 3.4	37.3 ± 3.5	36.6 ± 3.6
MCV (fL)	67.4 ± 1.9	53.9 ± 1.2	45.6 ± 1.3	45.6 ± 1.0	47.8 ± 0.9	44.5 ± 1.8	43.1 ± 1.5	45 ± 5.2	46 ± 3.5	47 ± 3.4	47 ± 3.9
MCH (pg)	23.0 ± 0.6	18.8 ± 0.8	14.8 ± 0.6	13.9 ± 0.3	14.1 ± 0.2	13.7 ± 0.4	13.5 ± 0.4	—	—	—	—
MCHC (%)	34.5 ± 0.8	33.0 ± 0.5	31.9 ± 0.6	30.9 ± 0.5	29.5 ± 0.4	31.3 ± 0.9	31.6 ± 0.8	32 ± 2.0	33 ± 3.3	34 ± 3.0	36 ± 3.1
Total WBC (×10³/µL)	9.67 ± 0.57	15.31 ± 1.21	17.45 ± 1.37	18.07 ± 1.94	23.68 ± 1.89	23.20 ± 3.36	19.70 ± 1.12	15.9 ± 6.0	21.9 ± 6.8	18.3 ± 7.8	24.0 ± 12.5
Segmented neutrophils	5.96 ± 0.68	6.92 ± 0.77	9.57 ± 1.65	6.75 ± 1.03	11.00 ± 1.41	11.00 ± 1.77	9.74 ± 0.92	—	—	—	—
Band neutrophils	0.05 ± 0.02	0.11 ± 0.04	0.20 ± 0.06	0.22 ± 0.08	0.12 ± 0.09	0.15 ± 0.07	0.16 ± 0.07	—	—	—	—
Lymphocytes	3.73 ± 0.52	6.56 ± 0.59	6.41 ± 0.77	9.59 ± 1.57	10.17 ± 1.71	10.46 ± 2.61	8.78 ± 1.06	6.2 ± 2.1	5.3 ± 1.2	6.1 ± 2.0	5.5 ± 2.7
Monocytes	0.01 ± 0.01	0.02 ± 0.02	0	0.01 ± 0.01	0.11 ± 0.06	0	0.02 ± 0.02	—	—	—	—
Eosinophils	0.96 ± 0.43	1.40 ± 0.16	1.47 ± 0.25	1.08 ± 0.20	2.28 ± 0.31	1.55 ± 0.35	1.00 ± 0.19	—	—	—	—
Basophils	0.02 ± 0.01	0	0	0.02 ± 0.02	0	0.03 ± 0.03	0	—	—	—	—

Values in parentheses are mean values.
[a] Normal ranges ± one standard deviation from Meyers-Wallen VN, Haskins ME, Patterson DF. Hematologic values in healthy neonatal, weanling, and juvenile kittens. Am J Vet Res 1984;45:1322–7.
[b] Normal ranges from Anderson L, Wilson R, Hay D. Haematological values in normal cats from 4 weeks to 1 year of age. Res Vet Sci 1971;12:579–83.

Table 4
Puppy biochemical parameters from birth to approximately 8 weeks of age

	Days 1–3	Days 8–10	Weeks 4–5 Days 28–33	Weeks 7–8 Days 50–58
Albumin (g/dL)	1.76–2.75	1.71–2.5	2.17–2.97	2.38–3.22
ALP (U/L)	452–6358	195–768	153–490	153–527
ALT (U/L)	9.1–42.2	4.1–21.4	4.3–17.4	10.3–24.3
Bilirubin (mg/dL)	0.04–0.38	0.01–0.18	0.02–0.15	0.01–0.11
BUN (mg/dL)	29.5–118	29.1–66.7	13.1–46.2	16.8–61.4
Calcium (mg/dL)	10.4–13.6	11.2–13.2	10.4–13.2	10.8–12.8
Cholesterol (mg/dL)	90–234	158–340	177–392	149–347
Creatinine (mg/dL)	0.37–1.06	0.28–0.42	0.25–0.83	0.26–0.66
GGT (U/L)	163–3558	—	—	—
GLDH (U/L)	1.8–17.0	0.2–17.7	1.2–9.0	1.6–7.3
Glucose (mg/dL)	76–155	101–161	121–158	122–159
Total protein (g/dL)	3.7–5.77	3.26–4.37	3.71–4.81	4.04–5.33
Triglycerides (mg/dL)	45–248	52–220	36–149	39–120
Phosphorus (mg/dL)	5.26–10.83	8.35–11.14	8.66–11.45	8.35–11.14

Abbreviations: ALP, alkaline phosphatase; AST, aspartate aminotransferase; BUN, blood urea nitrogen; GGT, γ-glutamyltransferase; GLDH, glutamate dehydrogenase.
   Data from Refs.[8–10]

urinalysis. Low urine specific gravity (1.006–1.017) is normal, as is the detection of a small amount of protein, glucose, and various amino acids. By 3 weeks of age, urine protein and glucose concentrations approach those of an adult dog, and urine concentration is expected to compare with that of an adult dog by 6 to 8 weeks of age.[7]

Puppies and kittens may be more susceptible to drug toxicity because of their limited capacity to eliminate those drugs and drug metabolites that depend on renal excretory mechanisms. Antimicrobials, such as penicillins (ampicillin, β-lactams) and cephalosporins are usually the drugs of choice in young puppies and kittens. The author's preferred antimicrobial in the neonate is ceftiofur sodium (Naxcel, Pharmacia & Upjohn), 2.5 mg/kg subcutaneously every 12 hours for a maximum of 5 days due to its minimal effects on the intestinal flora and usual effectiveness against causative organisms. The potential for renal toxicity with nonsteroidal anti-inflammatory drugs (NSAIDs) in the neonate is far greater than in the adult animal, and their use in the neonate is generally not advised.

HEPATOBILIARY SYSTEM

During gestation, the maternal placental circulation supports the functionally immature hepatobiliary system of the fetus. In most dogs, the functional closure of the ductus venosus gradually occurs during the second and third days after birth. Complete morphologic closure of the ductus (which occurs as the ductus atrophies) is established by 1 to 3 months after birth.[14] Despite early embryogenic differentiation of the liver, many of its metabolic functions are incompletely developed at birth. The fetal liver has reduced capacities for gluconeogenesis, glycogen storage, bile acid metabolism, detoxification, and elimination processes, thus rendering it more susceptible to transplacental and postnatal toxic and infectious insults that may be inconsequential in adults.

Table 5
Puppy biochemical parameters up to 12 months of age

	2–3 Months	4–6 Months	7–12 Months
Albumin (g/dL)[a]	2.6–3.7	2.6–3.7	2.6–3.7
ALP (U/L)	88–532	126–438	4–252
ALT (U/L)	≤29	≤32	5–45
Amylase (U/L)[a]	≤1683	≤1683	≤1683
AST (U/L)	7–19	3–23	2–26
Bilirubin (mg/dL)	0.01–0.13	0.01–0.13	≤0.3
BUN (mg/dL)[a]	9.8–37.3	9.8–37.3	9.8–37.3
Calcium (mg/dL)	10.4–13.6	10–13.2	10.4–12
Chloride (mEq/L)[a]	99–120	99–120	99–120
Cholesterol (mg/dL)	99.6–499.6	99.6–499.6	135–278
CK (U/L)	31–255	40–192	≤134
Creatinine (mg/dL)	0.39–0.49	0.27–0.88	0.21–0.89
GGT (U/L)	≤6.2	≤4.3	≤3.2
Globulins (g/dL)	1.9–2.5	2.2–3.5	2.2–4.5
Glucose (mg/dL)	97.1–166.2	97.1–166.2	76–119
GLDH (U/L)	1.6–9.6	1.9–8.7	1.2–8.0
LDH (U/L)	68–290	≤442	9–269
Lipase (U/L)	≤241	≤139	≤154
Magnesium (mEq/L)[a]	1.4–5.2	1.4–5.2	1.4–5.2
Phosphorus (mg/dL)	6.4–11.3	5.6–9.6	3.5–7.8
Potassium (mEq/L)	4.5–6.3	3.9–6.1	4.2–5.6
Sodium (mEq/L)	140–156	139–159	138–158
Total protein (g/dL)	4.3–5.8	4.5–7.3	4.9–6.7
Triglycerides (mg/dL)	19.1–205.5	19.1–205.5	40–169
TLI (µg/L)	5–35	—	—

Abbreviations: CK, creatine kinase; LDH, lactate dehydrogenase; TLI, trypsin-like immunoreactivity.
[a] Parameters for which significant age variation was not found in puppies.
Data from Refs.[10,15–19]

Normal values for routinely used biochemical indicators reflecting the status of the hepatobiliary system in newborn and growing puppies and kittens are given in **Tables 5–7**.

Neonatal puppies possess overall poor glycemic regulation compared with adults. Their inability to recovery quickly from either hypoglycemia or hyperglycemia may be attributed to a relative insensitivity to endogenous insulin and suboptimal counterregulatory hormone responses. Symptomatic hypoglycemia is uncommon in neonatal cats, and may reflect their carnivore-based metabolism.[14] Maintaining euglycemia is also vital for the neonatal neurologic status. Neonates have a relative deficiency of alternative energy sources (such as fat stores, gluconeogenic amino acids) compared with adults. Although glucose regulation improves with age, puppies and kittens up to 4 months of age should be considered predisposed to hypoglycemia when anorexic or dehydrated.

The neonate's capacity for hepatic uptake, conjugation, and excretion of bilirubin is remarkably mature. Information on the capacity of the feline neonatal hepatobiliary system is lacking. Some puppies and kittens demonstrate mildly elevated total

Table 6
Kitten biochemical parameters from birth to 8 weeks of age

	Day 0	Day 1	Day 7	Week 4 Day 28	Week 8 Day 56
Albumin (g/dL)	2.5–3.0	1.9–2.7	2.0–2.5	2.4–4.9	2.4–3.0
ALP (U/L)	184–538	1348–3715	126–363	97–274	60–161
ALT (U/L)	7–42	29–77	11–76	14–55	12–56
Amylase (U/L)	310–837	310–659	187–438	275–677	407–856
AST (U/L)	21–126	75–263	15–45	15–31	14–40
Bilirubin (mg/dL)	0.1–1.1	0.1–1.6	0.0–0.6	0.0–0.3	0.0–0.1
BUN (mg/dL)	26–45	34–94	16–36	10–22	16–33
Calcium (mg/dL)	9.4–13.9	9.6–12.2	10.0–13.7	10.0–12.2	9.8–11.7
Cholesterol (mg/dL)	65–141	48–212	119–213	173–253	124–221
CK (U/L)	91–2300	519–2654	107–445	125–592	102–1512
Creatinine (mg/dL)	1.2–3.1	0.6–1.2	0.3–0.7	0.4–0.7	0.6–1.2
GGT (U/L)	0–2	0–9	0–5	0–1	0–2
Glucose (mg/dL)	55–290	65–149	105–145	117–152	94–143
LDH (U/L)	176–1525	302–1309	117–513	98–410	62–862
Lipase (U/L)	12–43	21–131	8–46	4–86	6–70
Phosphorus (mg/dL)	5.9–11.2	4.9–8.9	6.7–11.0	6.7–9.0	7.6–11.7
Total protein (g/dL)	3.8–5.2	3.9–5.8	3.5–4.8	4.5–5.6	4.8–6.5
Total solids (g/dL)	3.1–4.4	3.2–5.2	3.0–4.6	4.0–6.0	4.1–6.2
Triglycerides (mg/dL)	23–132	30–644	129–963	43–721	16–170

Data from Levy JK, Crawford PC, Werner LL. Effect of age on reference intervals of serum biochemical values in kittens. J Am Vet Med Assoc 2006;228(7):1033–7.

bilirubin values and icteric serum during the first 72 hours of birth, but this usually resolves within 2 weeks in dogs, and up to 4 weeks of age in cats.[14] The etiology of this anomaly remains unclear.

Reference-range intervals for serum liver enzyme activities are essential for interpreting laboratory data in neonatal puppies and kittens. Differences in serum enzyme activity between neonates and adults reflect the decreased functional capacity of the liver, trauma associated with birthing, colostrum ingestion, maturation of metabolic pathways, growth effects, and differences in volume of distribution, body composition, and nutrition. Activity of serum alkaline phosphatase (ALP), aspartate aminotransferase (AST), γ-glutamyltransferase (GGT), creatinine kinase (CK), and lactate dehydrogenase (LDH) usually markedly increase during the first 24 hours of life.[14] These profound elevations usually persist 10 to 14 days postpartum, and decrease to moderate levels after 2 weeks of age. In kittens, ALP, CK, and LDH activity exceeds adult values through 8 weeks of age, whereas AST increases only transiently after birth. ALP remains above the adult reference range in cats and dogs, and usually stabilizes at adult reference ranges between 1 and 2 years of age. The source of the ALP and GGT activity is likely attributed to placental, colostral, and/or intestinal origin.[8]

The function of the urea cycle matures at varying stages of fetal and neonatal development in different species. Baseline ammonia levels values in clinically normal dogs and cats as young as 2 months have been demonstrated to be within the adult reference range, with the exception of some Irish Wolfhounds with the delayed closure of the ductus venosus.[14]

Table 7 Kitten biochemical parameters up to 12 months of age			
	<3 Months	4–6 Months	7–12 Months
ALT (U/L)	10–50	≤77	≤85
ALP (U/L)	≤564	37–333	21–197
Amylase (U/L)[a]	≤1800	1800	≤1800 (≤2200 Oriental breeds)
AST (U/L)	≤20	≤30	≤30 (≤40 Oriental breeds)
Bilirubin (mg/dL)[b]	≤4	≤4	≤4
BUN (mg/dL)[c]	17–35	17–35	17–35
Calcium (mg/dL)[a]	9.2–12.0	9.2–12.0	9.2–12.0
Chloride (mEq/L)	97–125	102–122	104–124
Creatinine (mg/dL)	0.16–1.26	0.33–1.21	—[d]
CK (U/L)	≤188	≤160	≤128
GGT (U/L)[a]	≤4	≤4	≤4
GLDH (U/L)[a]	≤7	≤7	≤7 (≤16 Oriental breeds)
Glucose (mg/dL)[c]	70–150	70–150	70–150
LDH (U/L)	68–280	≤442	9–269
Lipase (U/L)	≤280	≤280	≤280
Magnesium (mEq/L)[a]	1.2–5.2	1.2–5.2	1.2–5.2
Potassium (mEq/L)	3.7–6.1	4.2–5.8	3.7–5.3
Phosphorus (mg/dL)	6.5–10.1	6–10.4	4.5–8.5
Sodium (mEq/L)[a]	143–160	143–160	143–160
Total protein (g/dL)[e]	—	3.3–7.5	3.3–7.5
TLI (μg/L)	17–49[f]	—	—

[a] Parameters for which significant age variation has not been found in kittens.
[b] Adult values reached after 1 week of age.
[c] Adult values reached after 8 weeks of age.
[d] Reference ranges have not been reported for kittens older than 6 months; 0.8–2.3 mg/dL (adult).
[e] Adult levels are reached between 6 months and 1 year of age.
[f] Data from Refs.[16,17,20,21]

The utility of serum bile acids (SBA) for the assessment of liver function and perfusion has been fully investigated in neonatal, juvenile, and adult dogs and cats. SBA concentrations in 1-day-old and 1-, 2-, and 4-week old puppies and kittens are within the adult reference range. In older puppies and kittens, paired SBA samples (preprandial and 2-hour postprandial) concur with the adult reference range.[14]

Liver function is also responsible for the synthesis of albumin, cholesterol, many globulins, most coagulation, and many anticoagulant factors. Total protein and albumin concentrations in young dogs up to 4 weeks of age are below normal adult ranges, whereas protein concentrations in cats are more variable. By 8 weeks of age, puppies have normal adult albumin concentrations, whereas total serum globulin values increase with age, likely reflecting ongoing antigenic stimulation. Total protein concentration gradually increases to achieve adult levels within 6 months to 1 year of age. Coagulation assessments are limited in neonates, but seem to fall within the normal adult reference ranges for prothrombin time (PT), activated partial thromboplastin time (APTT), and fibrinogen in animals as young as 8 weeks of age.[14] Mild hypocholesterolemia is common in 1- to 3-day-old puppies but not kittens. In puppies and kittens older than 2 to 4 weeks of age, serum concentrations are within the adult normal range.

Hepatic microsomal enzyme activities are demonstrated to be 85% of that present in an adult dog by 4 weeks of age. Adult levels of P450-specific activity are not observed until 4.5 months of age.[7]

Clinical Implications

ALP activity increases dramatically after suckling. In 1- to 3-day-old puppies, ALP activities are more than 30 times higher than adult values, primarily because of high levels of ALP in colostrum. The measurement of ALP in serum or plasma may provide some important information on the passive transfer status in puppies. ALP in kittens has also been shown to be a predictor of passive transfer of colostral antibodies in kittens. ALP concentrations higher than 1500 U/L on day 1 after birth and greater than 500 U/L on day 2 after birth are relatively sensitive and specific for predicting adequate colostral ingestion in kittens.[12] Similarly to ALP, GGT activities may be used as a surrogate marker of adequate colostrum ingestion in puppies, with values approximately 100 times higher than adult values; however, unlike in puppies, GGT has not been shown to be a useful predictor of passive transfer in kittens.

Virtually no antibodies are transferred to canine and feline fetuses in utero because of the type of placentation, and they are thus born immunologically immature. Puppies and kittens depend on colostral transfer of antibodies (passive transfer). Colostrum in puppies and kittens needs to be ingested within the first 24 and 16 hours of life, respectively. If a neonate is known not to have ingested colostrum, antibodies can be provided by administration of pooled serum or plasma from any vaccinated adult of the same species, given orally (if <12 hours old) or subcutaneously (within the first 24 hours). For puppies, maternal serum, pooled adult serum, or hyperimmune canine serum preparation can be administered. Hyperimmune canine serum may be purchased through certain regional veterinary blood banks. If the fetus is less than 12 hours old, one may administer 150 mL/kg body weight, divided, orally; or 50 mL/kg body weight subcutaneously, for 3 doses at 6- to 8-hour intervals in the puppy.[5,7,22] In the kitten, 15 mL (approximately 150 mL/kg) of pooled adult serum from several adults (mindful of blood type to prevent neonatal isoerythrolysis) can be administered subcutaneously, given as 3 boluses, administered at birth, then 12 and 24 hours later.[5,23-25]

Because of the absence of a fully developed microsomal and P450 enzyme activity in the neonate until 4 to 5 months of age, and the paucity of information regarding altered pharmacokinetics in canine and feline neonates, the use of medications that require hepatic metabolism or excretion must be exercised cautiously (ie, phenobarbital, diazepam, NSAIDs).

The use of established adult reference ranges for SBA to identify hepatic and hepatoportal circulatory dysfunction is of value in puppies and kittens as young as 4 weeks of age. The use of a paired sample (12–24-hour fasted sample and 2-hour postprandial serum sample) is recommended rather than a fasted random bile acid, owing to physiologic variables that may influence this test.

LIPIDS

Because of the neonatal liver's decreased capacity to synthesize triglycerides and cholesterol, neonates rely predominantly on dietary absorption of lipids. Nursing is an important source of lipids in neonates.

In puppies, cholesterol and triglyceride concentrations are highest at less than 8 weeks of age. After weaning, the concentrations gradually decrease but may peak again at age 5 to 6 months. After 6 months of age, values usually decline until adult levels are reached.

In kittens, cholesterol and triglyceride concentrations are highest in nursing kittens. After weaning, the concentrations begin to decrease to reach adult levels by approximately ate 9 to 12 months of age. The upper reference limits for triglyceride and cholesterol in nursing kittens have been reported as up to 963 mg/dL and 521 mg/dL, respectively. Certain lipoproteins, particularly low-density lipoprotein, are significantly lower in kittens younger than 20 weeks than in older kittens (9–12 months of age) presumably because of the increased uptake of cholesterol to meet the needs of growth (**Tables 5–7**).[12]

Clinical Implications

Lipid imbalances may occur in puppies and kittens. Hypolipidemia may result secondary to starvation or malnutrition (ie, poor nursing, agalactia), maldigestion or malabsorption of fats (ie, exocrine pancreatic insufficiency, lymphangiectasia, inflammatory bowel disease), or liver dysfunction (ie, portosystemic shunt, infectious disease, toxic insult, hypoxemia).

Primary/congenital hyperlipidemia has been described in dogs and cats. Hyperchylomicronemia, a suspected hereditary autosomal recessive condition in cats, may result in severe hemolytic anemia, weakness, peripheral neuropathy, and lipemia retinalis. A primary hypercholesterolemia with normotriglyceridemia has also been reported in certain breeds, such as Rottweilers and Doberman Pinschers.[12]

Congenital hypothyroidism is uncommon, but has been reported in both puppies and kittens. Clinicopathologic features include hypercholesterolemia, hypercalcemia, and mild anemia. Hypercholesterolemia results from decreased hepatic metabolism and decreased fecal excretion of cholesterol. Treatment of congenital hypothyroidism in puppies and kittens is similar to the treatment of adult animals, using thyroid supplementation.

MINERALS

Calcium and phosphorus are important for proper bone growth but also for normal cell stability, muscle contraction, and acid-base regulation. Calcium and phosphorus levels are higher in young puppies and kittens throughout their growth phase. The presence of parathyroid hormone–related peptide and growth hormone in the milk during lactation also enhance calcium and phosphorus absorption in the neonate.

Calcium is highest in puppies younger than 8 weeks, and decreases to adult levels at about 1 year of age. Kittens also have higher calcium concentrations, relative to adult levels, before 8 weeks of age. However, unlike puppies, the calcium concentrations in kittens decrease shortly thereafter to reach adult levels by 3 months of age.[12]

Phosphorus concentrations are lowest at 1 to 3 days of age in puppies, then increase to above adult levels throughout the growth phase. Adult levels are reached at about 1 year of age. Kittens demonstrate their highest phosphorus concentrations when younger than 8 weeks, gradually decreasing to adult levels after 1 year of age.[12,13]

Clinical Implications

Decreased intake of dietary calcium and phosphorus is the most common cause of hypophosphatemia and hypocalcemia in young animals. Poor nutrition as a result of anorexia, poor nursing, or agalactia may all contribute to decreased mineral levels. Decreased vitamin D ingestion also contributes to the hypophosphatemia deficiency by leading to decreased phosphorus absorption.

Some additional causes of hypocalcemia in young animals include renal disease, ethylene glycol toxicosis, hypoalbuminemia, and metabolic alkalosis. Most causes of hypercalcemia are related to nutritional imbalances or renal dysfunction (ie, vitamin D toxicosis, congenital renal disease, granulomatous disease, and metabolic acidosis).

Decreased production of growth hormone is an uncommon congenital defect in pituitary development identified in several dog breeds, including German Shepherds, Spitz, and toy Pinschers, and may result in hypophosphatemia caused by decreased renal absorption of phosphorus.

REFERENCES

1. Bird KE. The hematologic and lymphoid systems. In: Peterson ME, Kutzler MA, editors. Small animal pediatrics: the first 12 months of life. St Louis (MO): WB Saunders; 2011. p. 305–27.
2. Clinkenbeard KD, Cowell RL, Meinkoth JH, et al. The hematopoietic and lymphoid systems. In: Hoskins JD, editor. Veterinary pediatrics: dogs and cats from birth to six months. 3rd edition. Philadelphia: WB Saunders; 2001. p. 300–43.
3. Chastain CB. The metabolic system. In: Hoskins JD, editor. Veterinary pediatrics: dogs and cats from birth to six months. 3rd edition. Philadelphia: WB Saunders; 2001. p. 359–70.
4. Davidson AP. Approaches to reducing neonatal mortality in dogs. In: Concannon PW, England G, Verstegen J III, et al, editors. Recent advances in small animal reproduction. Ithaca (NY): International veterinary information services; 2003; A1226.0303.
5. Kustritz MV. History and physical examination of the neonate. In: Petersen ME, Kutzler MA, editors. Small animal pediatrics: the first 12 months of life. St Louis (MO): WB Saunders; 2011. p. 20–7.
6. Kutzler MA. Causes of canine neonatal morbidity and methods to prevent losses. In. Proceedings of the LAVECCS. Distrito Federal (Mexico), July 12–15, 2012.
7. Grundy SA. Clinically relevant physiology of the neonate. In: Davidson AP, editor. Veterinary clinics of North America: small animal practice; pediatrics. Philadelphia (PA): W.B. Saunders; 2006. p. 443–56.
8. Center SA, Randolph JF, ManWarren T, et al. Effect of colostrum ingestion on gamma-glutamylaminotransferase and alkaline phosphatase activities in neonatal pups. Am J Vet Res 1991;52(3):499–504.
9. Kuhl S, Mischke R, Lund C, et al. Reference values of chemical blood parameters for puppies during the first 8 weeks of life. Dtsch Tierarztl Wochenschr 2000;107: 438–43.
10. Harper EJ, Hackett RM, Wilkinson J, et al. Age-related variations in hematologic and plasma biochemical test results in Beagles and Labrador retrievers. J Am Vet Med Assoc 2003;223(10):1436–42.
11. Kruger JM, Osborne CA, Lulich JP, et al. The urinary system. In: Hoskins JD, editor. Veterinary pediatrics: dogs and cats from birth to six months. 3rd edition. Philadelphia: WB Saunders; 2001. p. 371–2.
12. Gorman ME. Clinical chemistry of the puppy and kitten. In: Peterson ME, Kutzler MA, editors. Small animal pediatrics: the first 12 months of life. St Louis (MO): WB Saunders; 2011. p. 259–75.
13. Johnston SD, Root Kustritz MV, Olson PN. The neonate- from birth to weaning. In: Ray Kersing, editor. Canine and feline theriogenology. 1st edition. Philadelphia: WB Saunders; 2001. p. 146–67.
14. Center SA. The liver, biliary tract and exocrine pancreas. In: Peterson ME, Kutzler MA, editors. Small animal pediatrics: the first 12 months of life. St Louis (MO): WB Saunders; 2011. p. 368–74.

15. Kley S, Tschudi P, Busato A, et al. Establishing canine clinical chemistry reference values for the Hitachi 912 using the international federation of clinical chemistry (IFCC) recommendations. Comp Clin Path 2003;12:106–12.
16. Kraft W, Hartmann K, Dereser R. Dependency on age of laboratory values in dogs and cats. Part 1: activities in serum enzymes. Tierarztl Prax 1995;23:502–8.
17. Kraft W, Hartmann K, Dereser R. Age dependency of laboratory values in dogs and cats. Part II: serum electrolytes. Tierarztl Prax 1996;24:169–73.
18. Laroute V, Chetboul V, Roche L, et al. Quantitative evaluation of renal function in healthy Beagle puppies and mature dogs. Res Vet Sci 2005;79(2):161–7.
19. Vajdovich P, Gaál T, Szilágyi A, et al. Changes in some red blood cell and clinical laboratory parameters in young and old beagle dogs. Vet Res Commun 1997; 21(7):463–70.
20. Steiner JM. Diagnosis of pancreatitis. Vet Clin North Am Small Anim Pract 2003; 33:1181–95.
21. Kraft W, Hartmann K, Dereser R. Age dependency of laboratory values in dogs and cats. Part III: bilirubin creatinine & proteins in serum. Tierarztl Prax 1996; 24:610–5.
22. Poffenbarger EM, Olson PN, Chandler ML, et al. Use of adult dog serum as a substitute for colostrum in the neonatal dog. Am J Vet Res 1992;52:1221–4.
23. Levy JK, Crawford PC, Collante WR, et al. Use of adult cat serum to correct failure of passive transfer in kittens. J Am Vet Med Assoc 2001;219:1401–5.
24. Miller E. Diagnostic studies and sample collection in neonatal dogs and cats. In: Bonagura JD, editor. Kirk's current veterinary therapy XIII. Philadelphia: WB Saunders; 1995. p. 26–30.
25. Rickard V. Birth and the first 24 hours. In: Peterson ME, Kutzler MA, editors. Small animal pediatrics: the first 12 months of life. St Louis (MO): WB Saunders; 2011. p. 11–9.

Pros, Cons, and Techniques of Pediatric Neutering

Margaret V. Root Kustritz, DVM, PhD

KEYWORDS

- Pediatric • Castration • Ovariohysterectomy • Gonadectomy

KEY POINTS

- Pediatric anesthesia and surgery are safe, with decreased surgery time and quick patient recovery.
- The primary benefit of prepuberal gonadectomy in bitches and queens is decreased incidence of mammary neoplasia later in life.
- Detriments associated with gonadectomy at any age include various cancers, orthopedic problems including anterior cruciate ligament injury, and obesity.

INTRODUCTION

Pediatric gonadectomy is defined as ovariectomy or ovariohysterectomy, or castration, at 6 to 16 weeks of age. Significant research has been done regarding benefits and detriments of gonadectomy surgery. The reader is referred to extensively referenced review articles for detailed information.[1-4] Much of the published research looks at the large populations of gonadectomized versus intact animals without regard for age at the time of gonadectomy. The few studies that have specifically addressed age have shown no significant differences in long-term behavioral or medical outcomes of dogs and cats spayed or castrated at less than 24 weeks of age in comparison with those gonadectomized later, with the exception of increased incidence of infectious disease in one group of dogs gonadectomized when young that had come from one specific source.[5,6]

This article focuses on anesthetic and surgical techniques and what is known regarding timing of gonadectomy, especially regarding performance of these surgeries in pediatric dogs and cats. It is important to remember that association between many of the disorders described and gonadectomy is not necessarily an indication of cause and effect, and that other factors, including breed, environment, and body condition, may play a role. These factors are not specifically addressed here.

Department of Veterinary Clinical Sciences, University of Minnesota College of Veterinary Medicine, 1365 Gortner Avenue, St Paul, MN 55108, USA
E-mail address: rootk001@umn.edu

Vet Clin Small Anim 44 (2014) 221–233
http://dx.doi.org/10.1016/j.cvsm.2013.10.002
0195-5616/14/$ – see front matter © 2014 Elsevier Inc. All rights reserved.

ANESTHESIA AND SURGERY

Gonadectomy is an elective procedure, and should not be performed on animals that are not healthy and are not well able to tolerate anesthesia. The vaccination series need not be complete if the animal has received colostrum. All puppies and kittens should receive a complete physical examination and should be treated for internal parasites and, if necessary, for external parasites, before surgery.

Puppies and kittens tolerate anesthesia and surgery well, with quick recovery time. In one study evaluating student completion of ovariohysterectomy and castration surgeries in dogs and cats aged 8 to 16 weeks compared with animals older than 6 months, surgery times for cat spays, dog spays, and dog castrations were decreased by 6%, 29%, and 85%, respectively.[7] With completion of pediatric surgeries, students reported increased confidence in pediatric anesthesia and pediatric surgeries of all types, and improved general surgical skills.[8]

Concerns specific to anesthesia of pediatric animals include stress, hypoglycemia, hypothermia, and appropriate use of anesthetics and anesthetic equipment in physically small animals.[9] To minimize stress, it is recommended that pediatric animals remain housed in groups until induction of anesthesia, and that the induction area be as calm and quiet as possible. Pediatric animals have relatively little muscle mass with consequently smaller glycogen stores then adult animals, and have reduced capacity to raise blood sugar by glycogenolysis or gluconeogenesis because of immature hepatic function. Presurgical fasting time must be minimized, and the animal should be fed immediately on recovery.[10] Hypothermia occurs readily in pediatric animals because they have little body fat, a reduced ability to shiver to maintain their body temperature, and relatively greater surface area, permitting more rapid loss of body heat. Pediatric animals should be maintained on a warmed surface, preferably a warm-water circulating pad or similar diffuse heat source, from the time of induction through surgery and recovery. Surgical preparation liquids should be warmed before being applied to the animal.[11]

Studies evaluating induction time and quality, analgesia, maintenance of anesthetic depth, and recovery time and quality have proposed optimal anesthetic protocols for pediatric animals (**Table 1**).[12,13] There are published protocols using only inhalant anesthesia; these are not recommended because of the protracted excitation phase in animals induced by a mask, and because sufficient analgesia is not provided.

Table 1	
Optimal anesthesia protocols for spay-castration of puppies and kittens	
Species/Gender	**Optimal Anesthesia Protocol**
Canine, male	Propofol (6.5 mg/kg IV) 15 min after atropine (0.04 mg/kg IM) and oxymorphone (0.22 mg/kg IM). Use of midazolam (0.22 mg/kg IM) and butorphanol (0.44 mg/kg IM) instead of oxymorphone produced less sedation but good analgesia
Canine, female	Propofol (3.4 mg/kg IV) 15 min after atropine (0.04 mg/kg IM) and oxymorphone (0.11 mg/kg IM). Intubation-inhalant for maintenance
Feline, male	Tiletamine-zolazepam (11 mg/kg IM)
Feline, female	Midazolam (0.22 mg/kg IM) and ketamine (11 mg/kg IM). Intubation-inhalant for maintenance

Abbreviations: IM, intramuscular; IV, intravenous.
Data from Goeree G. Pediatric neuters can be technically challenging. Can Vet J 1998;39:244; and Faggella AM, Aronsohn MG. Evaluation of anesthetic protocols for neutering 6- to 14-week-old pups. J Amer Vet Med Assoc 1994;205:308–14.

Surgical techniques for ovariectomy and ovariohysterectomy are the same as for adult animals. It is not uncommon to find a significant volume of serous intra-abdominal fluid on laparotomy (**Fig. 1**).[11] Care should be taken in handling and stretching friable pediatric tissues.[12] The ovarian vessels and uterine vessels and body may be ligated with suture material or with hemostatic clips. The linea alba may be closed with either absorbable or nonabsorbable suture material. Closure of the skin with absorbable suture material in a subcuticular pattern may minimize self-trauma at the incision site.[12] Use of tissue glue to close the skin is discouraged, as there may be insufficient cohesion of tissues.[11]

Both testes usually are descended into the scrotum by 12 to 14 weeks of age in dogs and by birth in cats. Because the inguinal canal does not close until about 6 months of age in dogs and 7 to 8 months of age in cats, and because there is greater anesthetic and surgical risk associated with removal of a retained testis than a descended testis, it may behoove veterinarians to defer surgery and wait for testicular descent rather than to perform surgery in a young animal that requires laparotomy for complete castration.

Castration in cats is performed as in adult animals. Tying of the spermatic cord onto itself is discouraged because the spermatic cord is short and the tissues are friable.[11] Castration in very young puppies may be performed as in cats, with bilateral scrotal incisions and healing of incisions by second intention, or may be performed with a prescrotal incision and subcuticular closure with absorbable suture material, as in adult dogs.[12]

BENEFITS OF GONADECTOMY
Societal

The primary societal benefit of gonadectomy, and the primary reason veterinarians perform pediatric gonadectomy in dogs and cats, is population control.[14] It is currently estimated that 5 to 7 million dogs and cats enter humane societies yearly in the United States, and that approximately 3 to 4 million are euthanized.[15] Pediatric gonadectomy is more commonly performed at humane organizations than at veterinary practices, largely for reasons of population control. Historically, only about 50% to 60% of those adopting animals from humane organizations have had their animal spayed or castrated despite subsidizing the cost. Gonadectomy performed before adoption ensures that those adopted animals will not repopulate their shelter with their offspring, may

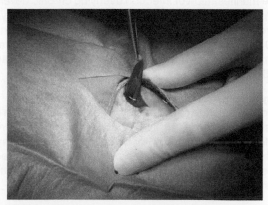

Fig. 1. Ovariohysterectomy in a puppy. Note small size of the uterine horn and ovary, and presence of serous fluid. (*Courtesy of* MN Spay Neuter Assistance Program, Plymouth, MN; with permission.)

increase adoptability of those animals, and increase retention of the animals in their adoptive homes.[14]

Behavioral

It is not difficult to hypothesize the effects of gonadectomy on behavior. Gonadectomy is associated with changes in neurosteroid biosynthesis in the brain.[16] Testosterone, estrogen, and progesterone are reported to have an anxiolytic effect, perhaps through stimulation of release of oxytocin and opioids; this effect may be lost with gonadectomy.[17–19]

Reproductive behaviors are decreased by performance of gonadectomy, with females showing no behavioral changes associated with estrus, and males showing less roaming, mounting, and urine marking (dogs) and urine spraying and sexual aggression (cats). Changes in urine-spraying behavior in both male and female cats also are affected by environmental factors, including other cats in the household and similar stimuli.[20,21] Gonadectomy will not effect change in inappropriate behaviors that are not driven by testosterone or estrogen (eg, fear-based aggression).

Medical

Mammary neoplasia

For female dogs and cats, the greatest benefits are decreased risk of development of mammary neoplasia when aged and lack of development of pyometra. Incidence of mammary neoplasia in cats is 2.5% and is virtually always malignant adenocarcinoma.[22–24] Mammary neoplasia is 7 times more likely to occur in aged queens than in spayed female cats, with the greatest decrease in incidence associated with spaying before the first estrus.[24] Incidence of mammary neoplasia in dogs is 3.4%, with about 50% being benign fibroadenomas and 50% malignant adenocarcinomas.[22,25–32] Incidence is greatly decreased by spaying, especially by spaying before the first heat.[1,33,34] A recent attempt to determine the significance of these data by systematic review of the veterinary literature was unable to identify strong evidence suggesting that spaying decreases the risk of mammary cancer; however, this systematic review is based on work in human medicine and requires a massive body of literature, which does not exist in veterinary medicine.[35]

Pyometra

Pyometra, an acute manifestation of infection overlying chronic development of cystic endometrial hyperplasia and exacerbated by endometrial reactivity under the influence of progesterone, is common in aged bitches, with a reported incidence of 23% to 25% by 10 years of age, and also occurs in queens.[36,37] Ovariohysterectomy at the time of diagnosis is curative, but mortality with surgical management is 0% to 17% in dogs and 8% in cats.[38,39]

Benign prostatic hypertrophy

With increasing age, the prostate of male dogs gradually increases in both cell number (hyperplasia) and size (hypertrophy). This process, termed benign prostatic hypertrophy (BPH), is manifested clinically in 50% of dogs by 2 to 3 years of age and in 75% to 80% by 6 years of age.[40–42] Castration is associated with loss of secretory epithelial cells and decrease in prostate size, with resolution of clinical signs.[43] The smaller prostate also is less likely to become infected.

Testicular neoplasia

Testicular neoplasia is a common neoplasm of aged dogs, with a reported incidence of 0.9%.[44] Three tumor types commonly are identified: Sertoli cell tumor, interstitial cell tumor, and seminoma. Metastasis is uncommon, and castration at the time of diagnosis is curative.

General considerations

In a large study of 1660 cats, gonadectomy before 5.5 months of age was associated with a decreased incidence of feline asthma in males and females, and a decreased incidence of abscesses, aggression toward the veterinarian, and urine spraying in male cats.[45] In a large study of 1842 dogs, gonadectomy at less than 5.5 months was associated with decreased frequency of episodes of separation anxiety and submissive urination.[46]

DETRIMENTS OF GONADECTOMY
Behavioral

Several behavioral changes have been associated with gonadectomy in dogs and cats. As mentioned earlier, behaviors not associated with testosterone or estrogen secretion are unlikely to be affected by gonadectomy. Some studies identified a greater number of aggressive dogs among gonadectomized populations, but these studies were done at humane organizations where it may well be that the dogs were gonadectomized in an attempt to control inappropriate behaviors and when this failed, were relinquished. Two differing types of behavior change have been specifically associated with gonadectomy. Increased reactivity and aggression have been identified in dogs after gonadectomy[47–51]; this may be associated with prior training or may be breed specific.[52,53] In one study, dogs castrated at less than 5.5 months of age were more likely to show aggression toward family members and strangers, and to bark excessively, in comparison with dogs castrated later in life.[46] Other studies refute these findings, with either no change in behavior or a decrease in aggressive behaviors noted with gonadectomy.[50,51,54–56] Cognitive decline was demonstrated to occur more quickly in one population of dogs after gonadectomy.[57] However, studies evaluating histologic changes in the brain associated with cognitive decline did not support gonadectomy as a causative factor.[58] In one survey of male and female cats gonadectomized at 6 to 13 weeks versus 6 to 7 months of age, no negative changes in behavior were noted.[59]

Questions regularly arise regarding changes in working ability of dogs after gonadectomy. In one study of male guide dogs, there were no differences in behavior or in placement rate as a working dog when comparing dogs castrated at 7 to 8 weeks, 6 to 8 months, or 10 to 14 months of age.[60] One publication describing management of dogs housed with flocks of sheep recommended castration, as it decreased premature death of those dogs caused by roaming with subsequent vehicular accidents, trapping, shooting, or poisoning.[61] Finally, one study evaluating effects of breed, gender, and intact status on trainability in dogs showed no effect of spaying on trainability of female dogs of any breed, no negative effect of castration in males of any breed, and a positive effect of castration on trainability of male dogs of one breed.[62]

Medical

Surgical complications
The complication rate after ovariohysterectomy has been reported as 6.1% to 27% in bitches and 2.6% to 33% in queens.[63,64] Intraoperative bleeding is of greatest concern in animals spayed while in estrus, and so is not a concern in prepuberal animals. Most complications are mild, not requiring veterinary intervention, and incidence is lower in young than in adult animals.[10,63]

Obesity

Retrospective surveys have consistently demonstrated increased body condition in dogs and cats after gonadectomy.[65,66] Research in rodents has shown an association between circulating steroid hormone concentrations and the concentration of adiponectin, a protein secreted by adipocytes that regulates lipid and glucose metabolism.[67] In cats, a decline in metabolic rate has been demonstrated after gonadectomy.[68,69] Other changes in cats postgonadectomy include increase in body weight of up to 20% greater than their initial weight, increase in insulin-like growth factor 1 and leptin, and increase in fasting glucose and triglyceride concentrations, suggesting profound changes in glucose metabolism.[70,71] In dogs, specific research documenting hormone changes and change in metabolic rate has not been published. Gonadectomy before 6 months of age was associated with a lower incidence of obesity in dogs in one study.[46] Obesity can be controlled by the animal's owner with appropriate diet and exercise.

Neoplasia

Incidence of several different types of cancers has been associated with gonadectomy in dogs, including prostatic carcinoma in male dogs, lymphosarcoma in male dogs, transitional cell carcinoma in female dogs, mast cell tumors in female dogs, and hemangiosarcoma and osteosarcoma in both male and female dogs. Cause and effect have not been defined. Because it also has been reported that life span is increased in animals that have been spayed or castrated, one might question whether this increased incidence is simply due to greater longevity in the gonadectomized population of dogs.[1]

Incidence of prostatic carcinoma in dogs is low, at 0.2% to 0.6%.[72,73] The reported increase in risk of developing prostatic carcinoma after castration is 2.4- to 4.3-fold.[72–75] Cause and effect are not defined.

Lymphosarcoma in golden retrievers was reported to be significantly more common in males castrated before 1 year of age than in intact males; no cases were reported in males castrated when older than 1 year of age in that study.[76] There is a breed risk for lymphosarcoma in golden retrievers, and cause and effect with gonadectomy are not defined.

Transitional cell carcinoma is reportedly more common in female dogs after ovariohysterectomy, with a 2- to 4-fold increase in risk.[77,78] Cause and effect are not defined.

Incidence of mast cell tumors was increased in female golden retrievers spayed after 1 year of age.[76] Cutaneous mast cell tumors were more common in spayed female dogs of various breeds than in intact female dogs.[79] Cause and effect are not defined.

Overall incidence of hemangiosarcoma, either of major vessels or the spleen, is 0.2% in dogs and 0.03% in cats.[1] Hemangiosarcoma was 4 times more common in female golden retrievers spayed after 1 year of age than in bitches spayed before 1 year of age or left intact in one study; in general, there is increased risk by a factor of 2.2 for splenic hemangiosarcoma and by a factor of 5 for cardiac hemangiosarcoma in spayed female dogs in comparison with intact bitches.[76,80,81] In male dogs, the overall risk of hemangiosarcoma is increased by a factor of 2.4 after castration.[80,81] Cause and effect are not defined.

Osteosarcoma is an uncommon tumor of dogs with high morbidity and mortality, with a reported incidence of 0.2%.[4] Gonadectomy is a risk factor, with a 1.3- to 2-fold increased risk reported.[82,83] Cause and effect are not defined.

Orthopedic problems

Injury or rupture of the cranial cruciate ligament has been reported to be more likely to occur in gonadectomized dogs than in intact dogs, even after accounting for the effect of obesity.[76,84–87] Cause and effect have not been identified, although hypothesized associations include changes in biomechanics resulting from hormonal change, and changes in structure of the stifle caused by alterations in growth-plate closure of the distal femur and proximal tibia, changing the tibial plateau angle and presumably putting more pressure on the cruciate ligaments. In rabbits, gonadectomy is associated with a decreased concentration of collagen in the cruciate ligaments.[88]

Canine hip dysplasia also is reported to be more common in gonadectomized than in intact dogs.[46,89] In a recent study of golden retrievers, the incidence of hip dysplasia was 10.3% in males castrated before 1 year of age compared with 5.1% in those left intact; no such effect of gonadectomy was demonstrated in female dogs in this study.[76] One hypothesized mechanism is alteration in hip-joint conformation caused by delays in physeal closure. In one study, although the incidence of hip dysplasia was higher in dogs gonadectomized when younger than 5.5 months, severity of disease was less than in dogs gonadectomized later in life.[46]

Closure of the growth plates of long bones depends on sex steroids. Growth-plate closure is delayed in dogs and cats that are gonadectomized prepuberally.[90–94] The clinical significance of this change is not known. Capital physeal fractures are reportedly more common in cats gonadectomized prepuberally, but obesity may have been a complicating factor in this study.[95]

General considerations
External genitalia of dogs and cats gonadectomized prepuberally is infantile compared with animals gonadectomized postpuberally or left intact.[91,96] Male cats castrated at 7 weeks of age were less likely to be able to extrude their penis from the prepuce in comparison with male cats castrated at 7 months of age or left intact.[96] The significance of these changes was not reported in these studies. It is hypothesized that maintenance of a juvenile vulva in female dogs, especially those who become overweight and have urinary incontinence, is associated with an increased incidence of perivulvar dermatitis and, perhaps, chronic vaginitis. In a large study evaluating long-term outcomes of dogs relative to age at gonadectomy, female dogs spayed before 5.5 months of age were more likely to develop cystitis, but none of the dogs described had more than 2 episodes of cystitis.[46]

Urinary incontinence, more specifically urethral sphincter mechanism incompetence, is more common in spayed than in intact female dogs, with an incidence of 5% to 20%.[97–100] In one large study, female dogs spayed at less than 3 months of age were at greatest risk; recent work refutes this, showing no correlation between age at gonadectomy and incidence of urinary incontinence.[46,97] A recent attempt to determine the significance of these data by systematic review of the veterinary literature was unable to identify strong evidence demonstrating an association between age at ovariectomy and onset of urinary incontinence; however, this systematic review is based on work in human medicine and requires a massive body of literature, which does not exist in veterinary medicine.[101] Specific cause and effect have not been defined, although it has been demonstrated that by 12 months after removal of ovaries, urethral closure pressure is significantly reduced.[102,103] This condition is more common in larger dogs than in small dogs.[97]

SUMMARY

There is much conflicting evidence in the veterinary literature regarding benefits and detriments of gonadectomy, with few of such studies directly addressing the effect of age at the time of surgery. One study asked veterinarians to rate morbidity and mortality of various disorders and multiplied this value by incidence to create an impact

Table 2
Impact[a] on health of male and female dogs after gonadectomy

Disorder	Female Dog	Male Dog	Female Cat	Male Cat
Mammary neoplasia	+24	—	+19	—
Pyometra	+100	—	—	—
Surgical complications	−20	−16	−7	−3
Osteosarcoma	−2	−2	—	—
Hemangiosarcoma	−2	−2	—	—
Transitional cell carcinoma	−7	−7	—	—
Prostate neoplasia	—	−3	—	—
Testicular neoplasia	—	+5	—	—
Urethral sphincter mechanism incompetence	−66	—	—	—
Benign prostatic hypertrophy	—	+368	—	—
Rupture of the cranial cruciate ligament	−11	−11	—	—
Obesity	−14	−13	−28	−26

[a] Positive impact score = benefit from gonadectomy; negative impact score = detriment from gonadectomy.

score, to help guide veterinarians as they educate clients or make decisions for stray animals in shelters (**Table 2**).[104]

For both species and genders, obesity is a significant detriment of gonadectomy. Veterinarians can use this opportunity to talk to clients about proper nutrition and exercise for maintenance of normal body weight. Setting aside obesity, the clear benefit of ovariohysterectomy for bitches and queens is evident. For male dogs, the high incidence of BPH artificially increases this impact factor. Because castration at the time of clinical manifestation of BPH is curative and because dogs are unlikely to develop clinical manifestations of this disorder until 2 to 3 years of age, castration can safely be deferred until that time in most dogs.[40–42] Benefits for male cats are primarily behavioral and are not readily assessed using impact factors. Because normal male cat reproductive behavior precludes their being good house pets and is readily controlled by castration, it is recommended that male cats be castrated prepuberally if they are not to be used for breeding.[105]

REFERENCES

1. Reichler IM. Gonadectomy in dogs and cats: a review of risks and benefits. Reprod Domest Anim 2009;44(Suppl 2):29–35.
2. Root Kustritz MV. Effects of surgical sterilization on canine and feline health and on society. Reprod Domest Anim 2012;47(Suppl 4):214–22.
3. Root Kustritz MV. Determining the optimal age for gonadectomy of dogs and cats. J Am Vet Med Assoc 2007;231:1665–75.
4. Root Kustritz MV. Optimal age for gonadectomy in dogs and cats. Clin Ther 2010;2:177–81.
5. Howe LM, Slater MR, Boothe HW, et al. Long-term outcome of gonadectomy performed at an early age or traditional age in dogs. J Am Vet Med Assoc 2001;218:217–21.
6. Howe LM, Slater MR, Boothe HW, et al. Long-term outcome of gonadectomy performed at an early age or traditional age in cats. J Am Vet Med Assoc 2000;217:1661–5.

7. Richardson EF, Gregory CR, Sucre E. Enhancement of the surgical education of fourth year veterinary students by participation in juvenile ovariohysterectomy and castration program [abstract]. Vet Surg 1994;23:415.
8. Howe LM, Slater MR. Student assessment of the educational benefits of a prepubertal gonadectomy program (preliminary findings). J Vet Med Educ 1997;24: 12–7.
9. Root Kustritz MV. Early spay-neuter in the dog and cat. Vet Clin North Am Small Anim Pract 1999;29:935–43.
10. Aronsohn MG, Faggella AM. Surgical techniques for neutering 6- to 14-week-old kittens. J Am Vet Med Assoc 1993;202:53–5.
11. Goeree G. Pediatric neuters can be technically challenging. Can Vet J 1998; 39:244.
12. Faggella AM, Aronsohn MG. Evaluation of anesthetic protocols for neutering 6- to 14-week-old pups. J Am Vet Med Assoc 1994;205:308–14.
13. Faggella AM, Aronsohn MG. Anesthetic techniques for neutering 6- to 14-week-old kittens. J Am Vet Med Assoc 1993;202:56–62.
14. Farnsworth MJ, Adams NJ, Seksel K, et al. Veterinary attitudes towards prepubertal gonadectomy of cats: a comparison of samples from New Zealand, Australia and the United Kingdom. N Z Vet J 2012. http://dx.doi.org/10.1080/00480169.2012.738591.
15. American Society for the Prevention of Cruelty to Animals. Pet statistics. Available at: http://www.aspca.org/about-us/FAQ/pet-statistics.aspx. Accessed March 21, 2013.
16. Ryzhavskii BY, Zadvornaya OV. Effect of gonadectomy on activity of neuronal 3β-hydroxysteroid dehydrogenase in some brain structures. Bull Exp Biol Med 2012;153:784–6.
17. Justel N, Ruetti E, Bentosela M, et al. Effects of testosterone administration and gonadectomy on incentive downshift and open field activity in rats. Physiol Behav 2012;106:657–63.
18. Mong JA, Pfaff DW. Hormonal and genetic influences underlying arousal as it drives sex and aggression in animal and human brains. Neurobiol Aging 2003;24:583–8.
19. Root Kustritz MV. Reproductive behavior of small animals. Theriogenology 2005; 64:743–6.
20. Hart BL, Cooper L. Factors relating to urine spraying and fighting in prepubertally gonadectomized cats. J Am Vet Med Assoc 1984;184:1255–8.
21. Rosenblatt JS, Aronson LR. The influence of experience on the behavioural effects of androgen in prepuberally castrated male cats. Anim Behav 1958;6: 171–82.
22. Dorn CR, Taylor DO, Frye FL, et al. Survey of animal neoplasms in Alameda and Contra Costa Counties, California. I. Methodology and description of cases. J Natl Cancer Inst 1968;40:295–305.
23. Verstegen J, Onclin K. Mammary tumors in the queen. Proceedings, Society for Theriogenology Annual Meeting. Columbus (OH), 2003. p. 239–45.
24. Hayes HM, Milne KL, Mandel CP. Epidemiological features of feline mammary carcinoma. Vet Rec 1981;108:476–9.
25. Dorn CR, Taylor DO, Schneider R, et al. Survey of animal neoplasms in Alameda and Contra Costa Counties, California. II. Cancer morbidity in dogs and cats from Alameda County. J Natl Cancer Inst 1968;40:307–18.
26. Fidler IJ, Brodey RS. The biological behavior of canine mammary neoplasms. J Am Vet Med Assoc 1967;151:1311–8.

27. Moe L. Population-based incidence of mammary tumors in some dogs breeds. J Reprod Fertil 2001;57:439–43.
28. Richards HG, McNeil PE, Thompson H, et al. An epidemiological analysis of canine-biopsies database compiled by a diagnostic histopathology service. Prev Vet Med 2001;51:125–36.
29. Cotchin E. Neoplasms in small animals. Vet Rec 1951;63:67–72.
30. Moulton JE, Taylor DO, Dorn CR, et al. Canine mammary tumors. Pathol Vet 1970;7:289–320.
31. Hampe JF, Misdorp W. Tumours and dysplasias of the mammary gland. Bull World Health Organ 1974;50:111–33.
32. Brodey RS, Goldschmidt MH, Roszel JR. Canine mammary gland neoplasms. J Am Anim Hosp Assoc 1983;19:61–90.
33. Schneider R, Dorn CR, Taylor DO. Factors influencing canine mammary cancer development and postsurgical survival. J Natl Cancer Inst 1969;43:1249–61.
34. Verstegen J, Onclin K. Etiopathogeny, classification and prognosis of mammary tumors in the canine and feline species. Proceedings, Society for Theriogenology Annual Meeting. Columbus (OH), 2003. p. 230–8.
35. Beauvais W, Cardwell JM, Brodbelt DC. The effect of neutering on the risk of mammary tumours in dogs—a systematic review. J Small Anim Pract 2012;53: 314–22.
36. Hagman R, Lagerstedt AS, Hedhammer A, et al. A breed-matched case-control study of potential risk-factors for canine pyometra. Theriogenology 2011;75: 1251–7.
37. Potter K, Hancock DH, Gallina AM. Clinical and pathologic features of endometrial hyperplasia, pyometra, and endometritis in cats: 79 cases (1980-1985). J Am Vet Med Assoc 1991;198:1427–31.
38. Johnston SD, Root Kustritz MV, Olson PN. Disorders of the canine uterus and uterine tubes (oviducts). In: Johnston SD, Root Kustritz MV, Olson PN, editors. Canine and feline theriogenology. Philadelphia: WB Saunders; 2001. p. 206–24.
39. Johnston SD, Root Kustritz MV, Olson PN. Disorders of the feline uterus and uterine tubes (oviducts). In: Johnston SD, Root Kustritz MV, Olson PN, editors. Canine and feline theriogenology. Philadelphia: WB Saunders; 2001. p. 463–71.
40. Zirkin BR, Strandberg JD. Quantitative changes in the morphology of the aging canine prostate. Anat Rec 1984;208:207–14.
41. Berry SJ, Strandberg JD, Saunders WJ, et al. Development of canine benign prostatic hyperplasia with age. Prostate 1986;9:363–73.
42. Lowseth LA, Gerlach RF, Gillett NA, et al. Age-related changes in the prostate and testes of the beagle dog. Vet Pathol 1990;27:347–53.
43. Al-Omari R, Shidaifat F, Dardaka M. Castration induced changes in dog prostate gland associated with diminished activin and activin receptor expression. Life Sci 2005;77:2752–9.
44. Hahn KA, VonDerHaar MA, Teclaw RF. An epidemiological evaluation of 1202 dogs with testicular neoplasia [abstract]. J Vet Intern Med 1992;6:121.
45. Spain CV, Scarlett JM, Houpt KA. Long-term risks and benefits of early-age gonadectomy in cats. J Am Vet Med Assoc 2004;224:372–9.
46. Spain CV, Scarlett JM, Houpt KA. Long-term risks and benefits of early-age gonadectomy in dogs. J Am Vet Med Assoc 2004;224:380–7.
47. Borchelt P. Aggressive behavior of dogs kept as companion animals—classification and influence of sex, reproductive status and breed. Appl Anim Ethol 1983;10:45–61.

48. Gershman K, Sacks J, Wright J. Which dogs bite—a case control study of risk factors. Pediatrics 1994;93:913–7.
49. Messam LL, Kass PH, Chomel BB, et al. The human-canine environment: a risk factor for non-play bites? Vet J 2008;177:205–15.
50. Podberscek AL, Serpell JA. Environmental influences on the expression of aggressive behavior in English spring spaniels. English Cocker Spaniels 1997;52:215–27.
51. Guy N, Luescher U, Dohoo S, et al. Demographic and aggressive characteristics of dogs in a general veterinary caseload. Appl Anim Beh Sci 2001;74:15–28.
52. Perez-Guisado J, Munoz-Serrano A. Factors linked to dominance aggression in dogs. J Anim Vet Adv 2009;8:336–42.
53. Reisner IR, Houpt KA, Shofer FS. National survey of owner-directed aggression in English Springer Spaniels. J Am Vet Med Assoc 2005;227:1594–603.
54. Hsu Y, Sun L. Factors associated with aggressive responses in pet dogs. Appl Anim Behav Sci 2010;123:108–23.
55. Van den Berg L, Schilder MB, De Vries H, et al. Phenotyping of aggressive behavior in Golden Retriever dogs with a questionnaire. Behav Genet 2006; 36:882–902.
56. Bennett PC, Rohlf VI. Owner-companion dog interactions: Relationships between demographic variables, potentially problematic behaviours, training engagement and shared activities. Appl Anim Behav Sci 2007;102:65–84.
57. Hart BL. Effect of gonadectomy on subsequent development of age-related cognitive impairment in dogs. J Am Vet Med Assoc 2001;219:51–6.
58. Waters DF, Shen S, Glickman LT. Life expectancy, antagonistic pleiotrophy, and the testis of dogs and men. Prostate 2000;43:272–7.
59. Wright JC. Early-age gonadectomy and the behavior of kittens reared in a household setting. Proceedings, Midwest Veterinary Conference. Columbus (OH), 2001.
60. DeSapio A, Van de Coevering P, Williams JD, et al. Effects of early-age gonadectomy on a male guide dog population. Proceedings, International Working Dog Breeding Conference. Melbourne (Australia), 2005.
61. Green JS, Woodruff RA. ADC guarding program update: a focus on managing dogs. Proceedings, Vertebrate Pest Conference. Sacramento (CA), 1990. Available at: http://digitalcommons.unl.edu/vpc14. Accessed March 20, 2013.
62. Serpell JA, Hsu Y. Effects of breed, sex, and neuter status on trainability in dogs. Anthrozoos 2005;18:196–207.
63. Romagnoli S. Surgical gonadectomy in the bitch and queen: should it be done and at what age? Proceedings, Southern European Veterinary Conference. Barcelona (Spain), 2008. Available at: http://www.ivis.org/proceedings/sevc/2008/romag1.pdf. Accessed March 18, 2013.
64. Pollari FL, Bonnett BN, Bamsey SC, et al. Postoperative complications of elective surgeries in dogs and cats determined by examining electronic and paper medical records. J Am Vet Med Assoc 1996;208:1882–6.
65. Courcier EA, Mellor DJ, Pendlebury E, et al. An investigation into the epidemiology of feline obesity in Great Britain: results of a cross-sectional study of 47 companion animal practices. Vet Rec 2012;171:560–4.
66. McGreevy PD, Thomson PC, Pride C, et al. Prevalence of obesity in dogs examined by Australian veterinary practices and the risk factors involved. Vet Rec 2012;156:695–702.
67. Yarrow JF, Beggs LA, Conover CF, et al. Influence of androgens on circulating adiponectin in male and female rodents. PLoS One 2012;10:e47315. http://dx.doi.org/10.1371/journal.pone.0043715.

68. Root MV, Johnston SD, Olson PN. Effect of prepuberal and postpuberal gonadectomy on heat production measured by indirect calorimetry in male and female domestic cats. Am J Vet Res 1996;57:371–4.
69. Fettman MJ, Stanton CA, Banks LL, et al. Effects of neutering on bodyweight, metabolic rate and glucose tolerance of domestic cats. Res Vet Sci 1997;62: 131–6.
70. Belsito KR, Vester BM, Keel T, et al. Spaying affects blood metabolites and adipose tissue gene expression in cats. Proceedings, Nestle Purina Nutrition Forum. St Louis (MO), 2007.
71. Martin LJ, Siliart B, Dumon HJ, et al. Spontaneous hormonal variations in male cats following gonadectomy. J Feline Med Surg 2006;8:309–14.
72. Bell FW, Klausner JS, Hayden DW, et al. Clinical and pathologic features of prostatic adenocarcinoma in sexually intact and castrated dogs: 31 cases (1970-1987). J Am Vet Med Assoc 1991;199:1623–30.
73. Teske E, Naan EC, Van Dijk EM, et al. Canine prostate carcinoma: epidemiological evidence of an increased risk in castrated dogs. Mol Cell Endocrinol 2002; 197:251–5.
74. Obradovich J, Walshaw R, Goulland E. The influence of castration on the development of prostatic carcinoma in the dog: 43 cases (1978-1985). J Vet Intern Med 1987;1:183–7.
75. Sorenmo KU, Goldschmidt M, Shofer F, et al. Immunohistochemical characterization of canine prostatic carcinoma and correlation with castration status and castration time. Vet Comp Oncol 2003;1:48–56.
76. Torres de la Riva G, Hart BL, Farver TB, et al. Neutering dogs: Effects on joint disorders and cancers in Golden Retrievers. PLoS One 2013;8:e55937. http://dx.doi.org/10.1371/journal.pone.005937.
77. Knapp DW, Glickman NW, DeNicola DB, et al. Naturally-occurring canine transitional cell carcinoma of the urinary bladder. A relevant model of human invasive bladder cancer. Urol Oncol 2000;5:47–59.
78. Norris AM, Laing EJ, Valli VE, et al. Canine bladder and urethral tumors: a retrospective study of 115 cases (1980-1985). J Vet Intern Med 1992;6:145–53.
79. White CR, Hohenhaus AE, Kelsey J, et al. Cutaneous MCTs: associations with spay/neuter status, breed, body size, and phylogenetic cluster. J Am Anim Hosp Assoc 2006;47:210–6.
80. Prymak C, McKee LJ, Goldschmidt MH, et al. Epidemiologic, clinical, pathologic, and prognostic characteristics of splenic hemangiosarcoma and splenic hematoma in dogs: 217 cases (1985). J Am Vet Med Assoc 1988;193:706–12.
81. Ware WA, Hopper DL. Cardiac tumors in dogs: 1982-1995. J Vet Intern Med 1999;13:95–103.
82. Priester WA, McKay FW. The occurrence of tumors in domestic animals. Natl Cancer Inst Monogr 1980;54:269.
83. Ru G, Terracini B, Glickman LT. Host related risk factors for canine osteosarcoma. Vet J 1998;156:31–9.
84. Amiel D, Ishizue KK, Harwood FL, et al. Injury of the anterior cruciate ligament: the role of collagenase in ligament deterioration. J Orthop Res 1989; 7:486–93.
85. Duval JM, Budsberg SC, Flo GL, et al. Breed, sex, and body weight as risk factors for rupture of the cranial cruciate ligament in young dogs. J Am Vet Med Assoc 1999;215:811–4.
86. Slauterbeck JR, Pankratz K, Xu KT, et al. Canine ovariohysterectomy and orchiectomy increases the prevalence of ACL injury. Clin Orthop 2004;429:301–5.

87. Whitehair JG, Vasseur PB, Willits NH. Epidemiology of cranial cruciate ligament rupture in dogs. J Am Vet Med Assoc 1993;203:1016–9.
88. Light VA, Montgomery RD, Akingbemi BT. Sex hormone regulation of collagen concentrations in cranial cruciate ligaments of sexually immature male rabbits. Am J Vet Res 2012;73:1186–93.
89. Van Hagen MA, Ducro BJ, Van Den Broek J, et al. Incidence, risk factors, and heritability estimates of hind limb lameness caused by hip dysplasia in a birth cohort of boxers. Am J Vet Res 2005;66:307–12.
90. May C, Bennett D, Downham DY. Delayed physeal closure with castration in cats. J Small Anim Pract 1991;32:326–8.
91. Salmerl KR, Bloomberg MS, Scruggs SL, et al. Gonadectomy in immature dogs: effects of skeletal, physical, and behavioral development. J Am Vet Med Assoc 1991;198:1193–203.
92. Houlton JE, McGlennon NJ. Castration and physeal closure in the cat. Vet Rec 1992;131:466–7.
93. Root MV, Johnston SD, Olson PN. The effect of prepuberal and postpuberal gonadectomy on radial physeal closure in male and female domestic cats. Vet Radiol Ultrasound 1996;38:42–7.
94. Stubbs WP, Bloomberg MS, Scruggs SL, et al. Effects of prepubertal gonadectomy on physical and behavioral development in cats. J Am Vet Med Assoc 1996;209:1864–71.
95. McNicholas WT, Wilkens BE, Blevins WE, et al. Spontaneous femoral capital physeal fractures in adults cats: 26 cases (1996-2001). J Am Vet Med Assoc 2002;221:1731–6.
96. Root MV, Johnston SD, Johnston GR, et al. The effect of prepuberal and postpuberal gonadectomy on penile extrusion and urethral diameter in the domestic cat. Vet Radiol Ultrasound 1996;37:363–6.
97. Forsee KM, Davis GJ, Mouat EE, et al. Evaluation of the prevalence of urinary incontinence in spayed female dogs: 566 cases (2003-2008). J Am Vet Med Assoc 2013;242:959–62.
98. Arnold S. Urinary incontinence in castrated bitches. Part I. Significance, clinical aspects and etiopathogenesis. Schweiz Arch Tierheilkd 1997;139:271–6.
99. Stocklin-Gautschi NM, Hassig M, Reichler IM. The relationship of urinary incontinence to early spaying in bitches. J Reprod Fertil 2001;57:233–6.
100. Angioletti A, DeFrancesco I, Vergottini M, et al. Urinary incontinence after spaying in the bitch: incidence and oestrogen therapy. Vet Res Commun 2004;28(Suppl 1):153–5.
101. Beauvais W, Cardwell JM, Brodbelt DC. The effect of neutering on the risk of urinary incontinence in bitches—a systematic review. J Small Anim Pract 2012;53:198–204.
102. Reichler IM, Pfeiffer E, Piche CA, et al. Changes in plasma gonadotropic concentrations and urethral closure pressure in the bitch during the 12 months following ovariectomy. Theriogenology 2004;62:1391–402.
103. Byron JK, Graves TK, Becker MD, et al. Evaluation of the ration of collagen type III to collagen type I in periurethral tissues of sexually intact and neutered female dogs. Am J Vet Res 2010;71:697–700.
104. Root Kustritz MV. Use of an impact score to guide client decision-making about timing of spay-castration of dogs and cats. Clin Ther 2012;4:481–5.
105. Hart BL, Barrett RE. Effects of castration on fighting, roaming, and urine spraying in adult male cats. J Am Vet Med Assoc 1973;163:290–2.

2013 Update on Current Vaccination Strategies in Puppies and Kittens

Gina M. Davis-Wurzler, DVM*

KEYWORDS

- Vaccination • Guidelines • Risk assessment • Puppies • Kittens

KEY POINTS

- Vaccines are perhaps one of the practitioner's greatest tools in preventing disease and maintaining individual and population health.
- Vaccines are to be used with forethought based on the risk of disease to the population and the individual, balanced with assessment of the risks associated with individual vaccines.
- It is the practitioner's role to educate pet owners regarding actual risks associated with both undervaccination and overvaccination.
- The goal is to reach the highest level of overall animal health with the minimum number of adverse events, based on scientific and epidemiologic merit.

This article is an update to "Current Vaccination Strategies in Puppies and Kittens" published in *Veterinary Clinics of North America, Small Animal Practitioner*, in May 2006. During her recent literature review as preparation for this update, the author has noted a significant increase in both interest and literature on this topic. There are now comprehensive guidelines readily available for small animal practitioners regarding canine and feline pediatric (and adult) vaccination recommendations. Perhaps more importantly, there is an increased dialogue regarding all aspects of preventive medicine, of which vaccination is only a small, yet significant portion; and an increased drive to provide scientific evidence for developing vaccination recommendations. The reader is strongly encouraged to read (and keep close at hand) the 2011 American Animal Hospital Canine Vaccination Guidelines and the 2013 American Associate of Feline Practitioners Feline Vaccination Advisory Panel Report (both readily available) for a sweeping review of vaccine types, indications,

Outpatient Medicine, Department of Veterinary Medicine and Epidemiology, School of Veterinary Medicine, University of California, One Garrod Drive, Davis, Davis, CA 95616, USA; Small Animal Outpatient Medicine Service, William R. Pritchard Veterinary Medical Teaching Hospital, Davis, CA 95616, USA
* Small Animal Outpatient Medicine, William R. Pritchard Veterinary Medical Teaching Hospital, Davis, CA 95616.
E-mail address: gmdavis@ucdavis.edu

Vet Clin Small Anim 44 (2014) 235–263
http://dx.doi.org/10.1016/j.cvsm.2013.11.006

recommendations, and adverse events; as such, a comprehensive discussion is not possible here. As veterinarians we should look forward to the ongoing growth of this area of interest within clinical practice and within the research community, to eventually provide practitioners with answers currently sought by pet owners and veterinarians alike.

It is far better to prevent than experience disease. This tenet should be the philosophy and goal of every veterinarian and every pet owner. For decades the veterinary profession has diligently educated pet owners about the benefits of preventing infectious disease, so well that there has been a significant decline in many of these diseases, in large part attributable to the development and use of effective vaccines. Veterinary practice staff members have done remarkable jobs sending reminder cards to ensure that canine and feline patients are current on their vaccinations. In fact, vaccines have become such a priority that many pet owners are inclined to forfeit other, indicated medical care in lieu of vaccines lest their beloved pets fall behind on their vaccine schedule. Veterinarians should commend themselves on a job well done, and commend pet owners for such conscientious stewardship of their pets. Now, however, the veterinary community must reflect on what has been accomplished, and make decisions for current and future patient care based on scientific, rational merit.

With the advent of knowledge on demand (ie, the Internet), pet owners have access to information regarding all issues of animal care. However, such information may not be accurate. It is our duty to educate pet owners; in fact, it should be seen as an opportunity. Who better to disseminate knowledge about veterinary medicine to the general public than veterinarians? No other group of individuals is as equipped with knowledge, skills, and insight as the veterinary community.

BASIC IMMUNOLOGY

To adequately discuss and understand how to make appropriate choices regarding pediatric vaccinations, a brief review and discussion of terms relative to basic immunology are warranted. Passive transfer of immunity occurs when maternal antibody is transferred by the dam or queen to the fetus via the placenta, which occurs minimally in dogs and cats. It also occurs during initial suckling through the ingestion of colostrum, which has more significant effects in these species.[1] This maternal immunity does provide initial protection against many pathogens, but of course depends on the health and immune status of the mother and the health of the fetus and neonate. Although this may result in temporary protection for the neonate, in the long term it may be deleterious to that individual's health by essentially keeping the animal naïve to different antigens (eg, maternal antibody interference with vaccination of the neonate). Maternal or passive immunization is effective in protecting neonates for the first several weeks of life, but begins to decline and lose the ability to protect against diseases rapidly as the maternal antibodies are degraded through natural catabolic processes. Between the ages of 6 and 16 weeks, depending on multiple factors (including species, amount of maternal antibody produced, transferred, and absorbed, and the individual health status of the neonate), most puppies and kittens have maternal antibody levels below protective levels. However, if present at high enough levels, maternal antibodies can interfere with the neonate's ability to respond to vaccination, as the circulating maternal antibody within the puppy or kitten may effectively respond to and neutralize the vaccine antigen, or render it ineffective by preventing recognition of the antigen by the immune system.[1] This is one reason why multiple, sequential vaccines are recommended in kittens and puppies until they are at least 14 to 16 weeks of age.[2,3] Of importance is that maternal antibodies can interfere with immunization, although the level of maternal antibody present may not be protective against pathogens.

A functioning immune system is composed of multiple parts. Innate immunity is the oldest (evolutionarily), least specific, and most immediate (in terms of response to potential invaders/pathogens) form of immunity. Macrophages, neutrophils, dendritic cells, and natural killer (NK) cells combined with numerous products produced by these cells comprise the innate immune system. Examples of some of the chemical components produced and released by these cells in response to microbial invasion include lysozyme, complement, various cytokines such as tumor necrosis factor α and interleukins, and various vasoactive molecules such as histamine.[4]

Active immunization is the process of the individual responding to an antigenic stimulus appropriately, by either natural infection or vaccination. Active immunization is processed through the acquired immune system. The 2 main types of acquired immunity are cell-mediated immunity and antibody, or humoral, immunity. Cell-mediated immunity is predominantly directed against pathogens that typically are obligate, intracellular organisms. Examples include viruses, some obligate intracellular bacteria, some fungi, and protozoa. T lymphocytes are the predominant effector cells, and depend on foreign protein (antigen) being presented to them before they can take effect against the pathogens; thus, multiple cell types are involved in forming cell-mediated immunity. Antibody or humoral immunity is predominantly directed against pathogens that can survive outside the host, or at least survive extracellularly. Examples include most bacteria, fungi, protozoa, and helminths. Multiple cells act in concert to confer humoral immunity as well, but the primary effector cell is the B lymphocyte.[5] Having stated this, in actuality humoral immunity is extremely important in protection against viral infections, and is intricately and definitively dependent on competent cell-mediated immunity.

Kittens and puppies will have varying degrees of ability to respond to antigens, whether resulting from natural or vaccine exposure, based on antigen load, route of exposure, antigenic virulence, genetics of the individual animal, and levels of persistent maternal immunity. In naïve animals whose maternal immunity has declined sufficiently so as not to interfere with an immune response; the first vaccine should stimulate a primary immune response (priming of the immune system). This initial exposure and recognition process and the ability to produce antibody to respond to the antigen typically takes 10 to 14 days; however, the maximum response takes up to 3 weeks. This primary response must not be confused with the animal having been immunized. A subsequent dose of vaccine (exposure) will lead to immunologic memory. Subsequent exposures to the same antigen elicit a stronger response: a greater amount of antibody is produced and the subsequent response is more rapid. This process is known as the secondary or anamnestic immune response, which results in immunity. Although multiple cell lines are involved in this response, subsets of T and B lymphocytes known as memory cells preserve the host's ability to recognize and respond to antigens to which the animal had previously been exposed.[4]

DEVELOPING VACCINE GUIDELINES USING RISK ASSESSMENT

To design, recommend, and actuate an effective plan for each patient, a practitioner must have familiarity with multiple variables. Those variables include duration of protection conferred on the neonate by the mother; the typical length of time maternal antibody may persist and pose interference with the young animal's ability to respond fully to a vaccine; and the length of time needed for an appropriate response. In addition, knowledge of the various diseases that pose risks to pediatric patients and knowledge of available safe, efficacious vaccines is critical. In essence, each patient must be assessed as an individual within the population to provide optimal wellness over the lifetime of each individual, as well as the population. This rationale has led to the concepts of core and noncore vaccines, 2 terms commonly used when discussing vaccination within the veterinary field. Criteria for assigning vaccines into these categories, and a third category, "generally not recommended," are based on: (1) morbidity and mortality associated with the specific disease (does the organism cause serious illness or does it cause a mild, transient disease that may pose only minimal risk to the individual or population?); (2) the prevalence and/or incidence rate of the disease (although a specific disease may not commonly be seen, the organism is ubiquitous in the environment and therefore poses risk to the individual or population); (3) the risk of the individual for exposure to the disease (indoor-only animal vs free-roaming individual, regional variations of occurrence); (4) the efficacy of the vaccine (does the vaccine prevent infection or simply ameliorate some signs or length of disease?); (5) the risks associated with administering the vaccine (are the risks associated with that vaccine greater than the risk of the disease?); (6) the potential for zoonotic disease; (7) the route of infection or transmissibility.[2,3,6–8] When these criteria are assessed, general guidelines may be generated for the individual practitioner and the veterinary community at large. Again, guidelines are not to be thought of as absolutes, nor are they to be used to establish standard of care. Simply stated, they are tools for each of us to use to promote optimal wellness for our patients when considering all factors affecting the individual's health (environmental, organismal [both pathogen and host], owner concerns, and current vaccine technologies).[2,3,6–8]

TYPES OF VACCINES

Multiple vaccines are available for canine and feline patients, although most fall within 3 basic categories. Assignment of vaccine products (which are considered biological agents, not drugs, and are therefore assessed and approved under the United States Department of Agriculture [USDA] Animal and Plant Health Inspection Service rather than the Food and Drug Administration) into these categories is based on how the product is created. Simply stated, modified live virus (MLV) vaccines are vaccines created by altering (attenuating) the pathogen in some way so that it is no longer able to cause serious or clinical disease in the targeted species. Killed vaccines are vaccines produced by inactivating the pathogen completely, rendering it incapable of reproducing and thereby unable to cause disease. The third category of vaccines consists of recombinant vaccines, of which there are multiple types, and this category itself has 3 subcategories. These vaccines use genetic technologies to either introduce genetic material directly into the host (no vector, eg, purified subunit vaccines or type I recombinant, is used), alter the genetic material to change its virulence (gene deletion, type II recombinant), or incorporate genetic material from the desired pathogen into an attenuated vector organism (eg, feline rRabies [r = recombinant], type III recombinant).[9,10] Within the near future, multiple new technologies are likely to provide even more choices, potentially providing patients with better protection against disease with minimal vaccine-associated risks. A more recent discussion for categorizing vaccines has evolved, and assigns vaccines to 1 of 2 groups: infectious or noninfectious. Simply stated, infectious vaccines include those biologics that have the ability to enter host cells and undergo replication within the host (ML, rCanary poxvectored vaccines). Noninfectious vaccines do not have the ability to undergo replication within the host.[3] For a comparison between vaccine types, the reader is referred to **Table 1**.

GENERAL RECOMMENDATIONS

Vaccines are available in single-dose and multiple-dose (tank) vials. The use of single-dose vial vaccines is highly recommended in these species. Conversely, the use of multiple-dose vials is discouraged because of the increased risk of contamination and the inability to assure consistent levels of antigen and adjuvant in individual doses from a single vial.[2,3] Multivalent vaccines are not recommended in cats other than the core feline vaccine designed to protect against feline panleukopenia, feline herpesvirus I, and feline calicivirus. Owing to increased inflammation at the site of multivalent vaccines, all other vaccines should be given as a separate vaccine, at the indicated site (see later discussion on feline core and noncore vaccines).[2,6] Allowing vaccines to acclimatize to room temperature before administration, particularly in cats, is recommended, as the administration of cold vaccines was found to have an increased association for tumorigenesis in cats.[11]

Use of sterile, single-use syringes is also recommended, as vaccines may become inactivated and/or ineffective with exposure to various products used to clean and sterilize syringes. Mixing of more than 1 vaccine within a syringe should not be performed because of the potential for inactivation of vaccine material, in addition to increasing the amount of antigen deposited within a single site. Moreover, administration of reconstituted vaccines (MLV r) should be done within 1 hour of reconstitution or otherwise discarded, owing to the potential inactivation of product and loss of efficacy.[3]

The practitioner is advised to always follow the manufacturer's directions for dose and route of administration. Using a topical product parenterally or splitting doses should never be done. A full dose is required to stimulate the immune system; there is no medical basis for giving a smaller dose to a toy breed dog, and this practice could lead to vaccine failure in that animal. If done with a rabies vaccine the practitioner is not following federal requirements, which carries potential legal implications.[3,12]

The interval between various vaccines, whether using the same product serially in the initial series or whether using different products in an adult animal, should never less than 2 to 3 weeks. Interference between the first product administered and a second vaccine product may lead to failure to optimally respond to the second vaccine. The exact mechanism of this interference is unknown, but may be associated with interferon produced by cells processing an MLV agent, or by transient immunosuppression by an MLV agent. Multiple vaccines administered at the same time do not appear to elicit this interference and is therefore an acceptable practice.[7,9] The reader is referred to **Tables 2** and **3** for comparison between pediatric canine and feline core, noncore, and generally not recommended vaccines.

CORE CANINE PEDIATRIC VACCINES

The diseases that fall within this category carry high rates of morbidity and/or mortality, are of public health concern, or are readily transmissible or may be ubiquitous in the environment. In addition, safe, efficacious vaccines are available and either provide sterile immunity (prevent infection) or confer a high degree of protection (do not prevent infection, but may confer protection such that the animal will not develop clinical signs of disease).[3,6] Essentially, the vaccines that fall within this category are recommended for each individual within the population regardless of the animal's lifestyle or locale.

Distemper

Canine distemper virus (CDV), an enveloped morbillivirus, has been well controlled because of the widespread vaccination programs over the last several decades. However, the disease still persists and, in addition to high virulence, it is readily

Table 1
Vaccine types, benefits, and associated concerns

Vaccine Type	Manufacturing Process, Method of Action	Associated Benefits and Recommendations	Associated Precautions and Contraindications
Modified live (attenuated)	Virus or bacteria made less virulent via cell or tissue passage. Attenuated viruses able to enter host's cells and replicate. Stimulates cell-mediated and humoral immunity	Mimics natural infection Rapid response by host's immune system Many products able to stimulate adequate immune response with a single dose Does not require use of adjuvant Vaccination of a single individual will lead to viral shedding, which may be useful in a herd-health situation when rapid exposure of multiple animals with an attenuated organism is desired	Potential to cause disease in some individuals (should not use in immune-compromised animals) Potential of organism to revert to more virulent form and cause disease even in healthy animals Special handling of vaccines required (temperature sensitive, shorter shelf life than killed products) Vaccinates shedding the modified live vaccinal organisms may lead to disease outbreaks in certain environments Parenteral administration of topical ML bacterin products may lead to serious disease (focal abscess at vaccine site, sepsis)
Killed (inactivated)	Virus or bacteria chemically or heat inactivated Organism unable to actively enter host's cells, unable to replicate Stimulates both cell-mediated and humoral immunity	No potential to revert to virulence Vaccinates do not shed the pathogen, therefore no potential to spread through population Indicated for use in immune-compromised animals (eg, FIV+ and FeLV+ cats) Organism does not cause disease in vaccinates Longer shelf life and less sensitive to temperature/handling requirements	Increased lag time of exposure to immune system leading to increased interval from vaccination to protection Because less immunogenic, these products require adjuvants (vaccine virus unable to actively enter host's immunocytes and replicate). Products containing adjuvants should be avoided in cats when alternative products with equal efficacy are available

	Terminology/Categorization	Advantages	Disadvantages
Recombinant (subunit, gene deleted, vectored)	Genetic material from pathogen altered in some way; 3 categories of recombinant vaccine technology use various techniques. Subunit vaccines are created by inserting specific genomic regions from the desired pathogen into nonpathogenic bacteria. The bacteria then produce protein as coded by the inserted genome. The desired protein is then harvested, purified, and used as a vaccine. Vectored virus vaccines incorporate immunogenic genomic regions from pathogen into an attenuated nonpathogenic virus	Vector able to penetrate host's cells, delivering genetic material from pathogen into the cell, therefore, no need for adjuvant. Rapid onset of immunity. Stimulates cell-mediated and humoral immunity. No potential for reversion to virulence. May be able to overcome maternal antibody interference earlier than modified live or killed products. Does not cause disease in healthy or immune compromised animals (appropriate for use in FIV+ and FeLV+). Vaccinates do not shed virus	Most killed products require a minimum of 2 doses to stimulate protective response. Greater potential for contamination and adverse reactions (require higher antigen load and adjuvants may cause adverse effects). Requires handling similar to modified live products (shorter shelf life, temperature sensitive). Increased cost in manufacturing and therefore increased cost to consumer
New (Alternative) Terminology/Categorization			
Infectious vaccine	Modified live/attenuated and canary pox-vectored recombinant vaccines	As stated above	
Noninfectious vaccine	Killed/inactivated (whole organism or particle), subunit vaccines	As stated above	

Abbreviations: FeLV, feline leukemia virus; FIV, feline immunodeficiency virus.

Table 2
Canine pediatric vaccines: core, noncore, and generally not recommended

Canine	Core	Noncore	Not Recommended
Distemper virus	MLV or recombinant beginning at 6–9 wk, given every 3–4 wk until ~16 wk old		
Adenovirus type 2 (CAV-II)	MLV, frequency as for CDV		
Parvovirus	MLV, frequency as for CDV		
Rabies	Killed, single dose, minimum age dependent on state and local regulations (12 or 16 wk)		
Leptospirosis		Killed bacterin, or purified subunit product, beginning at 12 wk, 2–3 doses given at 4-wk intervals	
Bordetella bronchiseptica		Attenuated bacterin, a single dose of an intranasal vaccine given 1 wk before potential exposure (minimum of 4 wk old)	
Parainfluenza		MLV, either use topical product combined with *B bronchiseptica* or parenteral vaccine contained in multivalent DAPP products	
Lyme disease (*Borrelia burgdorferi*)		Recombinant subunit vaccine (OspA) before exposure to ticks, 2 doses given 4 wk apart, beginning at 9 wk old	
Canine influenza		Killed-virus vaccine, typically not recommended but may be indicated in outbreak or kennel situations 2 initial doses 2–4 wk apart with first dose no earlier than 6 wk old	

(continued on next page)

Table 2 (continued)			
Canine	**Core**	**Noncore**	**Not Recommended**
Measles		Typically not recommended, use recombinant distemper vaccine for high-risk puppies instead of measles	
Coronavirus			Not recommended
Rattlesnake vaccine			Insufficient data to evaluate efficacy. Prevention of exposure, aversion training, and immediate veterinary attention postexposure highly recommended
Adenovirus type I (CAV-I)			Not recommended. CAV-II to prevent CAV-I infection is highly recommended

Abbreviations: CDV, canine distemper virus; DAPP, distemper, adenovirus 2, parvovirus, and parainfluenza; MLV, modified live virus; OspA, outer surface protein A.

transmissible. Infection with the virus causes respiratory, gastrointestinal, and neurologic signs, and is often fatal.[13] The distemper vaccine is commonly administered as part of a multivalent product. The general recommendation is to use a modified live or recombinant, multivalent product (CDV, canine adenovirus type II [CAV-II], canine parvovirus [CPV]) beginning at 6 to 9 weeks, and to give serial vaccines every 3 to 4 weeks until the puppy has reached 14 to 16 weeks of age.[3,9,14] Many studies support the improved ability of recombinant vaccines to overcome maternal antibody interference in comparison with modified live virus vaccines.[15,16] Most puppies will receive 2 or 3 distemper vaccinations, depending on the age at which they are first presented to the veterinarian. However, it is the interval between or the timing of the vaccinations, rather than the number, that is important. Serial vaccinations help to increase the likelihood of a complete response of the patient and thereby decrease the risk of vaccine failure that may occur when only 1 vaccine is administered. In addition, by eliciting a secondary immune response, they may help to increase the level of circulating antibody and decrease the lag time between exposure to an antigen and achievement of maximal antibody level.[4] Potential causes for vaccine failure include: a modified live vaccine that was improperly stored and therefore has lost its efficacy; the vaccine was improperly administered (wrong route or accidental loss of vaccine onto the skin of the patient); the patient's immune system did not respond (the immune system may have been responding to another antigenic challenge or the vaccine may have been given too soon after a previous vaccine); or maternal interference.[9] In theory, if a puppy were kept sequestered from exposure to this virus, 1 modified live distemper vaccine administered after 16 weeks of age would confer protection for at least 1 year.[1,3] However, in reality most pet owners are not inclined to isolate their puppies for the first 4 months of life, nor should they. Early socialization is an important part of families bonding with their puppies. Exposure to various people, other dogs, and new places helps decrease behavioral problems in the young adult and mature dog.[17] As long as the last distemper vaccine is administered after 16 weeks of age, the puppy should be able to mount a strong active response and fully overcome any residual maternal antibody. The current recommendation is to have the puppy return 1 year later (when approximately 16 months

Table 3
Feline pediatric vaccines: core, noncore, and generally not recommended

Feline	Core	Noncore	Not Recommended
Feline herpesvirus (feline viral rhinotracheitis)	MLV, give 2–3 doses of parenteral product beginning at 6–9 wk old, every 3–4 wk until ~12 wk old (or killed)		
Calicivirus	MLV, frequency as for FVR (or killed)		
Panleukopenia	MLV, frequency as for FVR		
Rabies	Recombinant canarypox-vectored product, single dose at minimum age of 12 wk but varies dependent on state and local regulations (or killed)		
Feline leukemia virus[a]	After viral screening confirming negative viral FeLV status, recombinant canarypox-vectored or killed product, 2 doses given 4 wk apart, as early as 8 wk old		
Chlamydiosis (Chlamydophila felis)			In high-risk environments, use parenteral attenuated bacterin product, 2 doses given 4 wk apart beginning at 9 wk old
Bordetella bronchiseptica			In high-risk environments, topical attenuated bacterin product designed for use in this species, single dose as early as 4 wk old
Feline immunodeficiency virus			Not generally recommended in kittens. Viral testing in kittens younger than 6 mo may yield false-positive results because of PMA. Vaccination causes positive Ab test
Feline infectious peritonitis			Not recommended. Vaccination causes positive Ab test

Abbreviations: Ab, antibody; FeLV, feline leukemia virus; FVR, feline viral rhinotracheitis; MLV, modified live virus; PMA, persistent maternal antibodies.

[a] Owing to increased susceptibility for infection in kittens, vaccination against feline leukemia virus is strongly recommended for all kittens. In single-cat households, households with known, negative viral status of all cats, and indoor-only cats, the practitioner may elect to consider this a noncore vaccine.

old) for another distemper vaccine. After the first annual vaccination, triennial immunization is recommended, regardless of vaccine type used.[2,3,9]

Canine Adenovirus

There are 2 types of adenovirus that cause disease in canine patients. Canine adenovirus type I (CAV-I), a nonenveloped virus in the family Adenoviridae, causes the potentially fatal disease infectious canine hepatitis. Clinical signs include fever, depression, vomiting and diarrhea, and potential petechiation and ecchymotic hemorrhage secondary to hepatic dysfunction. In addition, uveitis and renal disease are associated with infection with this virus. CAV-II causes respiratory tract disease. CAV-I is associated with severe, potentially fatal disease, and protection against this disease is recommended. Transmission is via the oronasal route and exposure to infected secretions. CAV-II infection typically results in mild self-limiting disease and is therefore considered to be a noncore disease; however, the modified live vaccine designed for prevention of CAV-I has been associated with adverse effects such as uveitis and corneal edema (an Arthus reaction, similar to effects caused by natural infection).[9,13] The current recommendation is to use the CAV-II modified live virus product, as it stimulates the immune system to protect against both CAV-I and CAV-II, without the associated adverse reaction caused by the type I vaccine.[3,14,18] The modified live adeno-type II virus is typically included in a multivalent injection (as mentioned earlier) and is therefore usually administered at intervals of 3 to 4 weeks, beginning between 6 and 9 weeks of age and ending between 14 and 16 weeks old. A vaccination 1 year later is recommended before instituting triennial vaccinations.

Canine Parvovirus

CPV is a nonenveloped type 2 parvovirus. The predominant form currently causing infection in the United States is type 2b, but other subtypes exist and cause disease elsewhere.[13] Because the virus is nonenveloped, it may exist (outside of a host) under certain environmental conditions, and is somewhat resistant to many disinfectants. Transmission is via the fecal-oral route, and clinical signs include lethargy, anorexia, pyrexia, vomiting, and diarrhea (typically hemorrhagic). Young animals appear to be at highest risk for developing severe, life-threatening disease. The current recommendation for vaccination is to use a multivalent MLV vaccine beginning at 6 to 9 weeks and to repeat the vaccine at intervals as already stated (every 3–4 weeks, until the puppy is 14–16 weeks old). In the past there was concern that certain breeds may have been at increased risk for contracting and developing severe parvoviral disease (Doberman Pinschers, Rottweilers), but it is generally agreed that these breeds will mount an appropriate response to a quality product if the last vaccine is given between 14 and 16 weeks of age.[3,13,19] There is, however, a small population of dogs that is genetically unable to respond to vaccination against CPV2, regardless of the number of vaccinations (nonresponders). One benefit of having a well-vaccinated population is that even those nonresponders are at decreased risk of exposure and subsequent infection by parvovirus, based on strong herd immunity. Studies using MLV CPV2b strains showed a higher antibody response to CPV2 and CPV2b, and were better able to overcome maternal antibody interference than the CPV2-strain vaccines used[20,21]; however, all CPV2 vaccines currently available should produce strong immunity in immunocompetent dogs. Immunization 1 year after completing the initial puppy series is recommended, with subsequent triennial vaccinations.[3,22,23]

There is also emerging evidence that Weimaraner puppies are at increased risk of developing a severe form of hypertrophic osteodystrophy (HOD) in association with vaccination with MLV distemper, adenoviral, and parvoviral products. The exact mechanism is unknown, but the current recommendation is to use killed products in this breed for their pediatric vaccinations, and consider starting vaccinations when they are slightly older.[12]

Rabies

Rabies virus, an enveloped virus in the rhabdoviridae family, is capable of infecting all mammals.[13] Because it is an enveloped virus, it is not stable in the environment and is readily inactivated by most common disinfectants. The virus is transmitted through infected saliva, most commonly from a bite by an infected animal. Clinical signs range from anxiety or other vague behavioral changes to pica, dysphagia, photophobia, and paralysis. Because of the zoonotic potential and implications regarding public health, canine vaccination programs are strongly regulated and enforced. The current recommendation is to vaccinate puppies using a killed-virus vaccine at a minimum of 12 or 16 weeks of age. State regulations vary as to the minimum age for canine rabies vaccination: in California the legal minimum age of canine vaccination against rabies is 16 weeks. A second rabies vaccine (killed product) is administered 1 year later and then annually or triennially thereafter, depending on local regulations.[3,6] It is the practitioner's professional responsibility for knowledge of and adherence to regional laws regarding rabies vaccination frequency.[24]

NONCORE CANINE PEDIATRIC VACCINES

Vaccines in the noncore category may have limited efficacy, or the organism causing disease is not readily transmissible or may have limited geographic distribution or prevalence. In addition, the diseases these vaccines are designed to prevent may be so mild or self-limiting that the risks associated with administering the vaccines may be greater than the actual disease. Lastly, some vaccines may interfere with common screening methods for disease detection, and are therefore not recommended unless absolutely warranted for a specific individual. It is the burden of the practitioner, along with the pet owner, to make decisions regarding which, if any, of the noncore vaccines should be administered to a puppy.[3,6–8]

Leptospirosis

A bacterial pathogen that causes acute hepatic and renal disease, leptospirosis is typically transmitted through urine of infected animals (reservoir hosts include dogs, rats, wildlife, and livestock), and in contaminated water. There are at least 2 different species (*Leptospira interrogans* and *Leptospira kirschneri*) that can infect dogs, with multiple serovars (variants of the same species) of *L interrogans* causing disease in dogs.[25] Although these organisms have the potential to cause serious disease, dogs are not likely to be at risk in a mostly urban, controlled environment (housed in a fenced yard with no exposure to wildlife or livestock). However, a dog that frequents rural environments or has exposure to waterways or livestock is definitely at risk of infection and should therefore be protected against the disease. Again, the initial puppy appointments should involve a through history and include the owner's plans for the dog's future use. If an owner brings a Labrador retriever puppy to the veterinarian for "whatever vaccines he needs," it is up to the practitioner to ask "will he be a hunting dog, will he be used in field trials, will he be exposed to wildlife and waterways?" The Border Collie who lives on a working sheep ranch surely should be vaccinated appropriately against leptospirosis. Conversely, a long-haired miniature Dachshund who will spend her days on her owner's lap in an urban setting will be at minimal risk of exposure and, therefore, vaccination is most likely not warranted.

In essence, regional distribution, seasonality (increased prevalence during and immediately following the rainy season), and lifestyle of the puppy will be factored into the decision as to whether the puppy should be vaccinated. If the decision is made to vaccinate against leptospirosis, the general recommendation is to wait until the puppy is at least 12 weeks old, at which time a killed or purified subunit vaccine is administered. Infection is serovar specific, and no cross-protection is seen between different serovars; therefore, vaccination with as many serovars known to cause disease in a given region is recommended. An initial series of 2 vaccinations should be administered 3 to 4 weeks apart and repeated at least annually thereafter, as long as the risk of exposure to the agent exists.[26] The recommendation to wait until the puppy is at least 12 weeks old before administering the leptospirosis vaccine is based on the increased potential for adverse events associated with killed vaccines, and to increase the likelihood of a complete immune response.[3,27]

Bordetella

Bordetella bronchiseptica is a bacterial agent that causes infectious tracheobronchitis. Infection with this agent may occur in concert with other agents infecting the respiratory tract (canine parainfluenza virus [CPiV], CAV-II). Transmission occurs via direct contact or through aerosolized microdroplets from infected dogs, and is most likely to occur under crowded conditions such as boarding and grooming facilities and dog-show venues. The current recommendation is to vaccinate puppies at risk a minimum of 1 week before potential exposure with a combination vaccine containing both an avirulent live bacterin for *B bronchiseptica* and a modified live CPiV. The vaccine can be administered to puppies as young as 3 to 4 weeks of age, but is generally not indicated unless the puppy is in a kennel environment.[27] Many organized puppy socialization and obedience classes commonly require proof of vaccination against *Bordetella* at the time of enrollment or before beginning the course. The general consensus is that intranasal vaccines are superior to parenteral vaccines, as they stimulate rapid local immunity (which is not affected by persistent maternally derived antibody).[6,9] Intranasal vaccines should never be given subcutaneously, owing to the potential for severe (in some cases fatal) reactions (**Fig. 1**). If the puppy will be intermittently exposed throughout the year (traveling to shows, boarding or grooming facilities) the vaccine should be repeated every 6 months to annually.

Parainfluenza

As already stated, CPiV may occur in concert with other respiratory tract agents. The vaccine recommendations are as stated for *B bronchiseptica* if indicated. There are

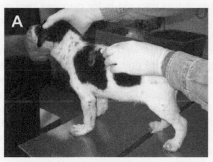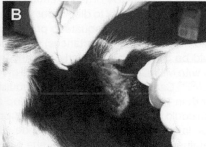

Fig. 1. (*A, B*) Local reaction with abscessation secondary to subcutaneous administration of a modified live bronchiseptica intranasal vaccine. (*Courtesy of* Dr Richard Ford, DVM, MS, DACVIM, Raleigh, NC.)

multiple products available, but the product currently recommended is the combination of intranasal vaccine containing a modified live parainfluenza virus with an attenuated *B bronchiseptica* bacterin. Intranasal vaccines can be used in puppies aged 3 to 4 weeks for individuals at high risk of exposure (depending on vaccine manufacturer label restrictions). For optimal protection, the vaccine should be administered every 6 months to annually if indicated. Alternatively many multivalent, parental products containing modified live CDV, CAV-II, CPV, and parainfluenza are available and appropriate for use.[3,9]

Borreliosis

Borrelia burgdorferi is a vector-borne, spirochete bacterium responsible for Lyme disease (borreliosis). Transmission occurs when an infected tick (various species within the *Ixodes* genera, also referred to as hard ticks) bites and remains attached to a host, in this case a puppy. Direct, horizontal transmission is not likely to occur, so the risk to humans and other pets is thought to be minimal. If a puppy has a significant burden with infected ticks, it of course increases the exposure to others in the household but, as ticks typically do not reattach once they have taken a complete meal, the risk is considered to be fairly small unless appropriate tick control is not instituted.[28] Vaccination to protect against Lyme disease is controversial, as the duration of immunity and degree of protection provided by vaccination is unknown, and vaccination with some vaccines interferes with standard screening diagnostics.[29] Therefore, vaccination against Lyme disease is warranted only if a puppy will be expected to be at high risk for tick exposure, and only if it lives in a *Borrelia*-endemic area. There are killed and recombinant (OspA subunit) vaccines available for use against *B burgdorferi*, and if vaccination is deemed warranted, the current recommendation is to use one of the subunit vaccines before exposure to ticks. The vaccine can be given as early as 9 weeks and should be repeated 3 to 4 weeks later.[27] The best prophylaxis is likely achieved by using appropriate tick prevention, such as fipronil with methoprene spray or spot-on products (eg, Frontline Top Spot; Merial Ltd, Iselin, NJ), amitraz collars (eg, Preventic collar; Virbac Animal Health, Fort Worth, TX), or an imidacloprid/permethrin topical product (eg, Canine Advantix; Bayer Animal Health, Shawnee Mission, KS).[29,30] These products should be chosen and recommended carefully by the veterinarian based on household situations, owner concerns, and the age of the puppy.

Measles

This virus, also a morbillivirus, can stimulate an immune response that is cross-protective against CDV. The indication for using this vaccine is for puppies that may have maternal antibody to distemper virus sufficient to cause interference with distemper vaccination but inadequate to protect against infection. If indicated (see later discussion on special circumstances), a single vaccination with a modified live vaccine should be given intramuscularly as early as 6 weeks of age. Subsequent immunizations with MLV CDV vaccines should be given serially as recommended (see CDV section).[1,3,31] Canine measles vaccines should never be administered to female puppies older than 12 weeks, as they may develop an acquired immune response to the virus, which could be problematic if a female puppy vaccinated against measles at 14 weeks of age later became pregnant. If she developed antibodies to the measles virus and maintained immunologic memory, she would confer measles antibody to her puppies via passive transfer, thus rendering measles vaccination in those puppies ineffective. A more appropriate alternative to administering a measles vaccine to a young puppy thought to be at risk for infection but too young to receive an MLV CDV vaccine would be to use a recombinant CDV vaccine, thereby decreasing the likelihood of maternal antibody interference.[3,32]

Canine Influenza Virus

Canine influenza virus has been seen in various countries, most notably in enzootic outbreaks. This virus is typically seen in puppies and dogs in shelter, boarding, and day-care facilities, and often occurs as a coinfection in canine infectious respiratory disease (CIRD) with bacterial pathogens. There is a commercially available inactivated vaccine available for use in puppies as young as 6 weeks. Vaccination with this product should be used only in puppies with a high risk of exposure, such as to shelters and areas known to be dealing with current/recent outbreaks (typically not in client-owned puppies). In addition, some countries now require an initial vaccination series (2 doses, given 2–4 weeks apart) before importation.[3,33]

Rattlesnake Vaccine

A vaccine designed to protect against envenomation by *Crotalus atrox*, the Western Diamondback rattlesnake, was released onto the market several years ago. The original provisional licensure was granted to provide possible protection against this single species of snake, and was granted for use only in California. The company was later granted extended licensure for multiple states, and has extended its claim for potential protection against multiple species of members of the Crotalidae (pit vipers). To date, no challenge studies have been performed in the canine species to validate efficacy claims. All claims are based on antibody titer to the venom component included in the vaccine, to murid challenge studies, and to field reports of protection of naturally occurring envenomation.[34] No controlled, independent studies exist concerning the impact of prior vaccination on therapeutics after envenomation. The manufacturer does not claim that vaccination with this product will completely protect against effects of envenomation; rather, they claim it may slow the onset of clinical signs and decrease the severity of signs. Immediate veterinary care is still the gold standard for any snake bite. Because of the great potential for variability in envenomation (site of bite on animal, size and age of snake, amount of venom injected into animal, and species of snake), field observations and anecdotal reports of protection are difficult to substantiate. Challenge studies conducted under controlled conditions will likely be necessary to validate the efficacy of this product. At present, owing to the preceding statements, this vaccine is not recommended for general use. Aversion training and keeping dogs out of areas known to favor rattlesnake habitation, and immediate veterinary evaluation and care are still the standard recommendations for preventing and treating disease associated with rattlesnake envenomation. If an owner is extremely concerned about the potential for exposure and envenomation by a Western Diamondback rattlesnake, the decision to vaccinate should be made after a discussion between the veterinarian and owner, with full disclosure of vaccine efficacy and a risk/benefit analysis, understanding the potential for adverse events from vaccination. This vaccine has been shown to be safe for use in puppies as young as 4 months.

CANINE, GENERALLY NOT RECOMMENDED
Canine Corona Virus

An enveloped virus belonging to the family Coronaviridae, this virus is transmitted via the fecal-oral route. Vaccination against this disease is generally not recommended because the vaccines provide questionable protection, and the actual prevalence and severity of the disease are unknown. Those most likely to be infected and develop clinical disease are neonates younger than 6 weeks. Clinical signs may include diarrhea, possibly hemorrhagic, but typically self-limiting. The general recommendation is to vaccinate puppies against CPV (as recommended in the section on CPV), as this practice appears to confer protection against coronavirus in addition to preventing infection with CPV2.[3,14]

Canine Adenovirus Type I

As stated in the canine core vaccine section, CAV-I causes serious disease in dogs; however use of the CAV-I is associated with a high incidence of adverse events. Vaccination with CAV-II induces an immune response that is protective against both CAV-I and CAV-II without the adverse effects. The recommendation is to use CAV-II as part of the canine core vaccination program; CAV-I should not be used.[3]

CORE FELINE PEDIATRIC VACCINES
Feline Panleukopenia Virus

Feline panleukopenia, a nonenveloped parvovirus closely related to canine parvovirus, causes serious, often fatal disease in kittens. Transmission typically occurs from direct contact with infected animals, although in utero infection and fomite transmission also occurs. Clinical signs typically include pyrexia, anorexia, lethargy, vomiting, and diarrhea. Kittens may be immunosuppressed subsequent to pancytopenia associated with this viral infection. Kittens infected in utero may exhibit cerebellar disease. Prevention is achieved by using modified live virus vaccines beginning between 6 and 9 weeks of age. The standard recommendation is to use a parenteral product (as opposed to intranasal products, which have higher incidences of postvaccinal viral shedding and potential for clinical disease induced by the more virulent viruses in these vaccines).[2,6,9] As is the case for canine distemper, adenovirus, and parvovirus, the core feline diseases, with the exception of rabies, are typically administered in a multivalent product in series. There are numerous vaccine products containing feline panleukopenia virus, herpesvirus I, and calicivirus (see later discussion). The current recommendation is to choose an MLV or killed product from a reputable manufacturer. Vaccines are administered subcutaneously in the distal aspect of the right thoracic limb (elbow or distally) and given every 3 to 4 weeks until the kitten is at least 16 to 20 weeks old. Repeat administration is recommended 1 year later before instituting a triennial schedule.[2,35]

Feline Herpesvirus I

Feline herpesvirus I (FHV-I), also known as feline viral rhinotracheitis virus, is an enveloped virus causing respiratory tract disease in cats. Clinical signs include sneezing, nasal congestion and discharge, conjunctivitis, and ocular discharge. In addition, kittens may exhibit pyrexia, anorexia, and lethargy along with oral/lingual ulcerations and associated hypersalivation. In some cases ulcerative, crusting dermatitis occurs, which may mimic other dermatologic disease.[36] The virus typically causes upper respiratory disease but the lower respiratory tract may become involved, especially in neonates or debilitated animals. Infection with this virus is lifelong, although many cats will "recover" and not show clinical signs. However, cats infected with FHV-I may have recurrent outbreaks, especially under times of stress or if their immunity is otherwise compromised. Cats may persistently shed the virus and act as a source of infection in shelters, catteries, and multiple-cat households. Therefore, prevention before exposure is key to controlling this disease.[36,37] Vaccination with a modified live virus (or killed product) beginning as early as 6 to 9 weeks is recommended, this being commonly administered as part of a multivalent product, given subcutaneously, in the right thoracic limb. The current recommendation is for kittens to receive a second vaccination 4 weeks later. The last vaccine in the series should be given when kittens are 16 to 20 weeks of age. A vaccine should be given 1 year later before beginning the triennial schedule.[2]

Feline Calicivirus

Feline calicivirus causes respiratory tract disease in kittens and cats. Because it is a nonenveloped virus, it is more resistant to disinfectants and may therefore persist in the environment. Signs are similar to those associated with FHV-I, but lameness and stomatitis are also commonly seen. Transmission of both FHV-I and calicivirus is through direct contact, exposure to contaminated secretions, aerosolization, and fomites.[36,37] Another, highly virulent, strain of feline calicivirus was identified several years ago and carries a higher incidence of mortality. Transmission is through either direct contact or via fomites. Prior vaccination against feline calicivirus does not appear to be protective against this strain, and adult cats appear to be more severely affected than kittens.[38,39] The current recommendation is as for panleukopenia and FHV-I: administering a modified live virus inactivated-virus parenteral vaccine beginning at 6 or 9 weeks with a subsequent vaccine 4 weeks later (the last vaccination should be when the kitten is at least 16 to 20 weeks old). A booster vaccine should be administered 1 year later, and then every 3 years.[2]

Rabies

As stated earlier, rabies virus affects all mammals and in the United States, with most documented cases of rabies in pet animals occurring in cats.[40] Because of the significant risk to pets, wildlife, and humans, vaccination against rabies virus is highly recommended for all kittens and cats, even those kept inside.[2,6] Local requirements vary, but the general recommendation is that all kittens should be vaccinated beginning at 12 weeks of age with either the recombinant rabies vaccine (preferable) or a killed rabies virus vaccine.[2,6,41] The recombinant product uses gene-splicing technology: reverse transcriptase is applied to rabies viral RNA to create complementary DNA. The segment of rabies virus DNA that codes (a codon) for the immunogenic protein associated with the virus (glycoprotein G) is then spliced from the rabies DNA and inserted into a canarypox virus. The canarypox virus, which is attenuated, is nonpathogenic to mammalian cells and therefore carries no potential to cause disease in this species. Because the vaccine is essentially a modified live product, the canarypox virus can enter cells, delivering the codon for rabies virus glycoprotein G to its targeted site. Once inside the cell the canarypox virus is unable to replicate, but the rabies glycoprotein G codon is preserved, leading the host cell to express the glycoprotein on its surface; this stimulates both cell-mediated and humoral immune responses. Besides the benefit of stimulating both types of immunity, because this product is adjuvant-free there may be a decreased risk of local inflammation associated with vaccination, thereby potentially decreasing the risk of subsequent vaccine reactions and tumorigenesis. The current recommendation is to use either the rRabies virus vaccine (preferred when possible) or a killed-virus vaccine in a case where increased duration of immunity is required (not pertinent to kittens because all pediatric/initial rabies vaccinations provide only 12 months of protection, regardless of label claims).[2,6] Rabies vaccines should be administered subcutaneously in the right pelvic limb, as distally as is reasonably possible: the level of the stifle is acceptable and areas distal to the tarsus are difficult to inject, and therefore not really feasible or appropriate. Administering vaccines (or any injections for that matter) in the tail should be avoided. Giving injections in the tail is difficult because of the scant amounts of loose skin and subcutaneous tissue, which is likely to cause more discomfort in patients during vaccination. More importantly, if a tumor does arise proximally on the tail, the potential for complete resection and cure are decreased because of the potential for tumor infiltration into the vertebral column. At present there is only one recombinant rabies vaccine approved for use in cats (PUREVAX Feline Rabies vaccine'; Merial Ltd, Duluth, GA). The current USDA approval/label states that this product should be administered annually. There are multiple killed-virus rabies vaccines approved for use in cats, with initial vaccination occurring at 12 weeks of age with a subsequent vaccination 1 year later. Because regulations vary depending on state or region, the veterinary practitioner must be familiar with local laws regarding rabies vaccination in this species.[24]

Feline Leukemia Virus

Feline leukemia virus (FeLV) is a retrovirus primarily affecting cats of any age, but kittens and juvenile cats appear to be most susceptible to infection.[42] Clinical signs are numerous and nonspecific, and include pyrexia, failure to thrive, chronic or recurrent respiratory tract, and gastrointestinal disease. Infection in kittens occurs via vertical transmission from the queen to the fetus, but may also spread horizontally from queen to kitten during lactation and grooming. Transmission also occurs through direct and usually prolonged contact with other infected cats from behaviors such as grooming and sharing food, and water bowls, and litter boxes. Viral screening using an enzyme-linked immunosorbent assay (ELISA) test designed to detect antigenemia should be performed on all kittens, even if their owners plan to house them strictly indoors. Because the ELISA test detects antigen, maternal antibody and vaccination do not interfere with test results. Therefore kittens of any age may be tested, and the current recommendation is to test every kitten (and adult cats with an unknown viral status) prior to FeLV vaccination.[43] If a kitten is antigen negative, the current recommendation is to administer either a killed or a recombinant vaccine on the first or second kitten visit. A second vaccine should be administered 4 weeks later followed by vaccination 1 year after the last FeLV kitten vaccine.[2,7] The recommended site for administration of any FeLV vaccine is the left pelvic limb, as distally as is reasonably possible.[2] At present there is only one recombinant FeLV vaccine available (PUREVAX Recombinant Leukemia vaccine; Merial Ltd, Duluth, GA). Although FeLV is considered a noncore vaccine in adult cats because kittens are most vulnerable to infection and may be exposed if outdoors, and immunity increases with age, it is rational to vaccinate all kittens against this disease with a repeat vaccination 1 year later. If the cat is subsequently housed strictly indoors and does not live with an infected (FeLV) cat, additional vaccinations are not indicated.[2]

NONCORE FELINE PEDIATRIC VACCINES
Chlamydiosis

Chlamydophila felis, formerly known as Chlamydia psittaci, is a bacterium that causes upper respiratory tract disease in kittens and cats. The most common sign is conjunctivitis, but sneezing and nasal discharge may also be present. Transmission is typically through direct contact with infected cats. Kittens are most commonly affected, but usually recover fully with appropriate antibiotic therapy: either topical oxytetracycline (Terramycin ophthalmic ointment) or systemic tetracycline (Panmycin Aquadrops) or doxycycline (Vibramycin). Vaccination against this agent typically does not prevent infection but may prevent clinical signs of disease. Because the vaccine does not fully prevent infection and carries an association with adverse events that may be greater than the actual disease, routine vaccination of household pets with this product is generally not recommended. However, it may be of use in some environments where the risk of infection is high, such as shelters or catteries with recent outbreaks.[2,44] If vaccination is deemed appropriate by the practitioner, an attenuated parenteral vaccine can be given to kittens beginning at 9 weeks, with a second dose given 3 to 4 weeks later.[45]

Bordetella

This bacterial agent causes respiratory tract disease in cats, and cats affected by stress, poor nutrition, or overcrowding seem more susceptible. Many kittens infected show mild, self-limiting disease with signs including pyrexia, sneezing, and nasal and ocular discharge, although bronchopneumonia has been documented. There is a topical, modified live bacterin vaccine designed for use in this species, but it is generally not recommended for routine use. If the practitioner feels protection against B bronchiseptica is warranted based on the kitten's risk of exposure, such as attendance at cat shows or visiting a boarding facility, or is in a shelter with potential contact with dogs (with a recent B bronchiseptica outbreak), administration of the vaccine designed for use in cats may be considered.[2] A single dose of the modified live intranasal vaccine can be given to kittens as young as 4 weeks of age.[2] The product designed for use in canines should not be used in cats.

FELINE, GENERALLY NOT RECOMMENDED

There are multiple vaccines in addition to those described and recommended here; however, many of these diseases pose a minimal risk to most of the feline population or the vaccines are minimally efficacious at preventing infection or disease, and therefore are generally not recommended. Additional reasons not to use some of these products are vaccine interference with screening tests and adverse events associated with some vaccines.

Feline Immunodeficiency Virus

A retrovirus, feline immunodeficiency virus (FIV) primarily affects cats by compromising their immune system, leaving them vulnerable to opportunistic infections. In addition to immunosuppression, with most of the effect targeted against the cell-mediated (T-cell) immune response, infection with FIV also carries an increased risk for development of certain types of neoplasia, B-cell lymphoma being the most common. Transmission occurs most commonly from breeding and fighting.[46] The virus is not spread through casual contact between housemates not engaging in the behaviors stated, nor is it spread through casual encounters between nonbreeding, non-fighting cats outside. Naturally occurring infection of kittens from queens is rare; however, kittens can become FIV-antibody positive via passive transfer from ingestion of colostrum of FIV-positive queens or queens previously vaccinated against FIV.[43,45] FIV-antibody levels acquired from maternal transfer in kittens who are actually FIV-virus negative decline over the first several months of life. The standard screening test for FIV is an ELISA test designed to detect FIV antibody. The ELISA was designed to detect antibody rather than antigen, because infected cats produce high levels of circulating antibody in contrast to low levels of circulating virus.[45] Because kittens may have circulating FIV antibody although actually may be FIV-antigen negative, it is generally not recommended to test kittens younger than 6 months. If a kitten is tested and a positive result is obtained, the test result should be repeated with a different methodology (Western blot or polymerase chain reaction [PCR]) and should be repeated once the kitten is more than 6 months old.[43] If a kitten is truly not infected, the maternal antibody will wane by 6 months of age, leading to seroconversion. If, however, a kitten or cat remains seropositive, the recommendation is made to keep the cat indoors only from that point, both to prevent infection of other cats and to decrease exposure to potential environmental pathogens. FIV-infected cats can live for years and, unless otherwise indicated by concurrent disease, euthanasia is generally not indicated for most owned pets. There is a killed FIV vaccine available, but the efficacy of this product is still unknown. There are 5 known subtypes of FIV virus, and the vaccine has been formulated to protect against subtypes A and D; however, the predominant subtype infecting cats in North America and Europe appears to be subtype B. It is unknown whether cross-protection exists between the different subtypes.[45] Because the vaccine elicits a strong antibody response, vaccinated kittens and cats will become seropositive on both ELISA and Western blot tests, as both tests detect antibody. A PCR test is available but is currently only performed at certain laboratories, and results and reliability vary with testing centers. Because of the increased technological needs and increased costs of this test, it is not considered the standard screening test. If done under specific conditions it can detect virus, and therefore may be of benefit in differentiating between cats with viremia (truly infected cats) and kittens or cats with circulating antibody, attributable either to maternal transfer or vaccination. Because of the nature of transmission of the virus and interference with the standard screening methods for infection, the vaccination against FIV is not currently recommended. Keeping cats indoors if possible, neutering all cats going outside, and preventing exposure to stray or feral cats that may be more likely to engage in fighting behaviors remain the gold standards for preventing this disease.[45,46]

Feline Infectious Peritonitis

The disease feline infectious peritonitis (FIP) is caused by a member of the Coronaviridae. Feline enteric coronavirus (FECV) and FIP virus are 2 phenotypes of the same virus. FECV transmission occurs through the fecal-oral route where it typically infects intestinal epithelium, but the organism can be transmitted via fomites and persists for long periods of time in the environment. Most cats infected with FECV either do not show clinical signs of disease or may have transient diarrhea, and some will persistently shed the virus in their feces.[47] FECV can, however, undergo random mutations within a host, creating FIP virus, although in most cats the virus does not mutate into this form and most cats will not develop FIP. The FIP virus enters and replicates within macrophages where it can then be disseminated throughout the body. Clinical signs are numerous, but commonly include weight loss, failure to thrive, diarrhea, pyrexia, and chronic respiratory tract disease. Two main types of the disease exist, the dry (noneffusive) and the wet (effusive) forms. Both are ultimately fatal diseases.[48] Although there is a vaccine available, its efficacy and indication for use is believed to be minimal, if at all.[48] The current recommendation is not to use this vaccine, based on efficacy concerns and the minimal risk of infection in most kittens and cats. Infection with FECV and mutation with subsequent development of disease occurs most commonly in multiple-cat households ($\geq$5), catteries, and shelters. The standard screening test for FIP is a serologic, indirect immunofluorescent antibody (IFA) test designed to detect antibody. This test may be of some value, but results need to be interpreted with caution, and concomitantly with signalment, clinical signs, and other laboratory data. Prior vaccination against FIP will yield positive IFA results, further posing potential complications in routing screening of this disease. In general, kittens are most vulnerable to this disease, with greater than 50% of cats with FIP being younger than 2 years.[48] Prevention is directed toward decreasing stress in kittens and cats in multiple-cat households, preventing exposure of naïve kittens and cats in environments known to have high endemic levels of feline enteric corona virus, and at depopulating catteries known to have high prevalence rates of FECV and FIP.[47,48] Because of the complexity of this disease and the limited space and objectives of this discussion, readers are encouraged to review *Infectious Diseases of the Dog and Cat*, 3rd edition, by Greene, and *Textbook of Veterinary Internal Medicine*, 7th edition, by Ettinger and Feldman, for a more comprehensive review of this disease.

ADVERSE EVENTS ASSOCIATED WITH VACCINES

Vaccines are potent biological agents designed to prevent disease. Any foreign product administered to an animal has the potential to be associated with an unexpected response by that animal. While vaccines must meet USDA requirements for safety, efficacy, potency, and purity, there still exists the potential for adverse events with products that have met these standards. Veterinarians should always report adverse events associated with vaccination to the vaccine manufacturer. Some adverse events are more likely to occur with certain agents, whereas others appear to have an increased rate of occurrence in certain breeds. Still others may be idiosyncratic and are not predictable. The following is offered as a brief overview of some types of adverse events associated with vaccination, with suggestions as to how a practitioner might best respond to and prevent such events from recurring.

The reactions seen most commonly are local inflammation at the site of the injection or general malaise, pyrexia, and anorexia for 1 to 2 days after vaccination.[12] Most of these reactions are self-limiting and require nothing more than monitoring by the animal owner. It is appropriate for the practitioner to note any reaction along with a description of signs documented in the medical record, and offer supportive care if indicated. In some instances administration of an MLV vaccine will cause transient mild clinical disease. Supportive care and isolation from unvaccinated animals is recommended, as the vaccinated animal showing clinical disease will shed the vaccinal organism and is potentially infectious to other animals.[9] Contact information for vaccine manufacturers, support agencies, and disease-reporting organizations is included in **Table 4**.

Feline Injection-Site Sarcomas

Feline injection-site sarcomas (FISS), formerly known as feline vaccine-associated sarcomas or fibrosarcomas, develop secondarily to local inflammation at injection sites. Originally it was thought that there was an increased risk for development of these tumors associated with specific adjuvants and vaccines; however, it is now accepted that all vaccines and repositol agents such as long-acting penicillin and corticosteroid injections, in addition to other injections, can be associated with the formation of FISS.[41] Measures to prevent these tumors are aimed at decreasing the local inflammatory response by avoiding the use of adjuvants in this species and administering only those vaccines indicated for the individual animal.[49,50] Multiple vaccines should not be administered in one site, as this may increase the amount of inflammation in that site. Following the recommended sites for injection is strongly recommended (see individual vaccine sections for specific sites)[2,6] and avoiding adjuvanted products when there is a reasonable alternative (MLV or recombinant) product available is ideal, as a recent study confirmed an increased association of tumor formation with adjuvanted vaccines compared with recombinant vaccines, although no vaccine was risk free.[51,52] There are specific guidelines as to how a practitioner should proceed if a cat develops a swelling at the site of a vaccine or injection. The practitioner is advised to monitor the patient closely, documenting 3-dimensional measurements and temporal association if a mass or swelling develops at the site of a vaccine. The 3-2-1 rule developed by the

Table 4
Support organizations, regulatory and disease reporting agencies, and vaccine manufacturers

Agency or Company	Address	Web Site and Phone Number	Support Available
American Animal Hospital Association	12575 West Bayaud Avenue, Lakewood, CO 80228, USA	www.aahanet.org 303.986.2800 Email: info@aahanet.org	Position statements on current vaccination guidelines, life-stage recommendations, standards for care and conduct
American Association of Feline Practitioners	390 Amwell Road, Suite 402, Hillsborough, NJ 08844, USA	www.catvets.com 800.874.0498	Position statements on viral screening, vaccination guidelines, life-stage recommendations, cat-friendly practice requirements
American Veterinary Medical Association	1931 North Meacham Road, Suite 100, Schaumburg, IL 60173-4360, USA	www.avma.org 800.248.2862	Links available to multiple sites, position statements on vaccination guidelines, zoonotic disease prevention and adverse event reporting (Feline Vaccine Sarcoma Task Force)
Centers for Disease Control and Prevention	1600 Clifton Road, N.E., Atlanta, GA 30333, USA	www.cdc.gov 800.CDC-INFO (800.232.4636)	United States government agency (department of Health and Human Services). Current information regarding infectious and noninfectious diseases

Center for Veterinary Biologics	USDA Animal and Plant Health Inspection Service	www.aphis.usda.gov 515.337.6100	Division of United States Department of Agriculture (USDA), contact agency for reporting adverse events associated with veterinary biologics
National Association of State Public Health Veterinarians, Inc	National Association of State Public Health Veterinarians	www.nasphv.org	Compendium of Animal Rabies Prevention and Control, rabies vaccination certificates available. List of all state veterinarians available online
Boehringer Ingelheim Vetmedica, Inc	3902 Gene Field Road, St Joseph, MO 64506, USA	www.boehringer-ingelheim.com Technical services: 800.325.9167	Manufacturer
Heska Corp	3760 Rocky Mountain Ave, Loveland, CO 80538, USA	www.heska.com 1.800.GO-HESKA (1.800.464.3752)	Manufacturer
Merck Animal Health	556 Morris Avenue, Summit, NJ 07901, USA	www.merck-animal-health-usa.com Companion Animal (dogs and cats): 800.224.5318	Manufacturer
Merial Ltd	3239 Satellite Blvd, Building 500, Duluth, GA 30096-4640, USA	www.merial.us Technical services: 1.888.MERIAL1, ext. 3 (1.888.637.4251, ext. 3)	Manufacturer
Virbac Corp	3200 Meacham Blvd, Ft Worth, TX 76137-4611, USA	www.virbacvet.com Technical services: 800.338.3659	Manufacturer
Zoetis	100 Campus Drive, Florham Park, NJ 07932, USA	www.zoetis.com 1.973.822.7000	Manufacturer

Feline Vaccine-Associated Sarcoma Task Force should be closely applied. "Three" refers to persistence of the mass for 3 months or greater; "2" refers to a size of 2 cm or greater; and "1" applies if the mass increases in size after 1 month. If any of these criteria are met, the mass should be biopsied with wedge technique or needle biopsy allowing for complete resection of the biopsy margins in the future, and subsequent referral to an oncologist or surgical oncologist if fibrosarcoma is confirmed. Fine-needle aspiration is not recommended for evaluation of potential injection-site sarcomas.[49,50] Most vaccine manufacturers have programs established to help defray the medical and surgical costs associated with these tumors, and the practitioner is advised to always notify the vaccine manufacturer any time an adverse event is seen.

Type I Hypersensitivity

Type I hypersensitivity, also known as immediate hypersensitivity and, in some cases, anaphylaxis, is mediated by immunoglobulin E antibody. The host's immune system may react to anything contained within the vaccine product, including cellular products used for culture, adjuvant, preservative, and the antigen itself, and reaction typically occurs within 2 to 3 hours after the administration of a vaccine. In the dog, signs range from urticaria, angioedema, and pruritus (**Fig. 2**) to respiratory distress and fulminant vascular collapse (anaphylaxis). In the cat, acute onset of vomiting and diarrhea with associated hypovolemia and respiratory and vascular shock may be seen.[12] If an animal develops any of these signs within the first several hours after vaccination, it should be presented to the veterinarian immediately for emergency medical care and support. It is not the goal of this review to offer therapies for shock, so the reader is referred to emergency veterinary literature for recommended therapies. The point here is to advise the practitioner to proceed with caution when using vaccines that may have a higher incidence of these reactions, or in breeds that may be at increased risk for immediate hypersensitivity. The increased association between killed bacterin vaccines and type I reactions is well documented, and there are reports that toy breeds may be at increased risk for type I reactions associated with these vaccines. If an animal does have a type I reaction to a vaccine, the signs shown by the patient, interval between vaccine and onset of signs, and therapeutics administered should be well documented in the medical record, as well as plans for future vaccination of the patient in question. Once an animal has this type of reaction to a vaccine, ideally the product should not be used again in that patient. All subsequent vaccines should be administered after a complete physical examination, and the vaccine should be given

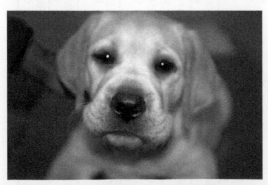

Fig. 2. Type I hypersensitivity (angioedema) in a Labrador retriever puppy after vaccination. (*Courtesy of* Dr Autumn Davidson, DVM, DACVIM, Davis, CA.)

early in the day to allow monitoring of the patient in the hospital for several hours. However, if this is not possible the patient should remain in the veterinary hospital for monitoring for at least 30 minutes followed by subsequent monitoring by the owner at home for several hours. Pretreatment with diphenhydramine (Benadryl) is an option, given parenterally (subcutaneous or intramuscular routes) at the dose of 1.0 mg/kg 15 to 30 minutes before vaccination if hypersensitivity is a concern. However, administration of corticosteroids concurrently with vaccination to prevent a hypersensitivity reaction is neither appropriate nor recommended because of potential immunosuppression and vaccine interference.[9] The patient's medical record should be identified, outside and inside, to prevent future accidental readministration of the product. Advising the owner that the patient should never receive that product again is important.

Type II Hypersensitivity

Type II hypersensitivity reactions (autoimmune reactions) are suspected to occur in dogs secondarily to vaccine administration. Although this theory is yet unproved, there are reports of dogs developing immune-mediated thrombocytopenia and immune-mediated hemolytic anemia temporally associated with recent vaccination. If a dog develops either of these conditions within 1 to 2 months after vaccine administration, the practitioner is advised to strongly consider the risk/benefit ratio of subsequent use of that product in the patient.[9,53]

Type III Hypersensitivity

Type III hypersensitivity reactions are immune complex reactions. Examples include the anterior uveitis associated with use of the CAV-I vaccine and the complement-mediated rabies vaccine induced vasculitis-dermatitis seen in dogs. Other examples include glomerulonephritis and polyarthritis. Antihistamine administered at the time of vaccine will do nothing to prevent the reaction, nor is it recommended to administer corticosteroids concurrently with vaccination. Once an animal has had this type of reaction, subsequent use of the product should be avoided in that patient.[9,54]

Type IV Hypersensitivity

Type IV hypersensitivity reactions are cell-mediated responses occurring locally or systemically. Examples include sterile granulomas at the sites of vaccine administration or polyradiculoneuritis. Many sterile granulomas resolve without any intervention, but for more severe reactions the practitioner is referred to various medicine texts for recommendations.[9,53]

SPECIAL CIRCUMSTANCES

The foregoing discussion applies mainly to puppies and kittens owned by individuals. Puppies and kittens housed in shelters face unique challenges, as do orphaned animals. These animals may not have received colostrum, and it is more likely that their mothers were not adequately vaccinated. The implications are that these animals are less likely to have received maternal antibodies, leaving them more vulnerable in the earliest stages of life. In addition, they frequently are malnourished, have an increased parasite burden, and are placed in crowded environments possibly with high numbers of endemic pathogens. The American Animal Hospital Association Canine Vaccination Task Force and American Association of Feline Practitioners have developed recommendations specifically designed for puppies and kittens in these environments. In general, neonates who may not have received colostrum or who are housed under the aforesaid conditions may be vaccinated at an earlier age, and ideally should be vaccinated before or at the time of entry into the shelter. Use of recombinant products may be of benefit in these animals, as well as additional vaccines (noncore vaccines). Husbandry is extremely important in these animals: providing proper nutrition, anthelmintics, and clean, dry housing is paramount. In general, these animals are special subsets of the general population facing challenges most young animals do not experience. Fiscal considerations and overall population health applies in these cases much more so than to individual, client-owned pets.

SUMMARY

Vaccines are perhaps one of the practitioner's greatest tools in preventing disease and maintaining individual and population health. Vaccination is to be used with forethought based on the risk of disease to the population and the individual, balanced with assessment of the risks associated with individual vaccines. It is the practitioner's role to educate pet owners regarding actual risks associated with both undervaccination and overvaccination. The goal is to reach the highest level of overall animal health with the minimum number of adverse events, based on scientific and epidemiologic merit.

REFERENCES

1. Tizard I. Immunity in the fetus and newborn. In: Veterinary immunology. 9th edition. St Louis (MO): Elsevier-Saunders; 2013. p. 225–39.
2. Scherk MA, Ford RB, Gaskell RM, et al. 2013 AAFP Feline Vaccination Advisory Panel report. J Feline Med Surg 2013;15(9):785–808.
3. American Animal Hospital Association Canine Vaccination Task Force, Welborn LV, DeVries JG, et al. 2011 AAHA canine vaccination guidelines. J Am Anim Hosp Assoc 2011;47(5):1–42.
4. Tizard I. The defense of the body. In: Veterinary immunology. 9th edition. St Louis (MO): Elsevier-Saunders; 2013. p. 1–10.
5. Tizard IB. Cells and their response to antigen. In: Veterinary immunology. 9th edition. St Louis (MO): Elsevier-Saunders; 2013. p. 150–64.
6. Klingborg DJ, Hustead DR, Curry-Galvin EA, et al. AVMA Council on Biologic and Therapeutic Agents' report on cat and dog vaccines. J Am Vet Med Assoc 2002;221(10):1401–7.
7. Ford RB. Vaccines & vaccinations: guidelines vs. reality. In: Proceedings of the American Board of Veterinary Practitioners Practitioner's Symposium 2005. Washington, DC, April 29-May 1, 2005.
8. Ford RB. Vaccines and vaccinations: the strategic issues. Vet Clin North Am Small Anim Pract 2001;31(3):439–53.
9. Greene CE, Schultz RD. Immunoprophylaxis. In: Greene CE, editor. Infectious diseases of the dog and cat. 3rd edition. St Louis (MO): Saunders Elsevier; 2006. p. 1073–7.
10. Tizard I. Vaccines and their production. In: Veterinary immunology. 9th edition. St Louis (MO): Elsevier-Saunders; 2013. p. 258–70.
11. Kass PH, Spangler WL, Hendrick MJ, et al. Multicenter case-control study of risk factors associated with development of vaccine-associated sarcomas in cats. J Am Vet Med Assoc 2003;223(9):1283–92.
12. Tizard I. The use of vaccines. In: Veterinary immunology. 9th edition. St Louis (MO): Elsevier- Saunders; 2013. p. 272–82.

13. Crawford PC, Sellon RK. Canine viral diseases. In: Ettinger SJ, Feldman EC, editors. Textbook of veterinary internal medicine, vol. 1, 7th edition. St Louis (MO): Elsevier Saunders; 2010. p. 958 Chapter 216.

14. Greene CE, Ford RB. Canine vaccination. Vet Clin North Am Small Anim Pract 2001;31(3):473–92.

15. Fischer L, Tronel JP, Pardo-David C, et al. Vaccination of puppies born to immune dams with a canine adenovirus-based vaccine protects against a canine distemper virus challenge. Vaccine 2002;20(29–30):3485–97.

16. Welter J, Taylor J, Tartaglia J, et al. Vaccination against canine distemper virus infection in infant ferrets with and without maternal antibody protection using recombinant attenuated poxvirus vaccines. J Virol 2000;74(14): 6358–67.

17. Hunthausen WK. Preventive behavioral medicine for dogs. In: Horwitz D, Mills D, Heath S, editors. BSAVA manual of canine and feline behavioural medicine. 2nd edition. Quedgeley (Gloucester): British Small Animal Veterinary Association; 2010. p. 65–6.

18. Greene CE. Infectious canine hepatitis and canine acidophil cell hepatitis. In: Greene CE, editor. Infectious diseases of the dog and cat. 3rd edition. St Louis (MO): Saunders Elsevier; 2006. p. 41–7.

19. McCaw DL, Hoskins JD. Canine viral enteritis. In: Greene CE, editor. Infectious diseases of the dog and cat. 3rd edition. St Louis (MO): Saunders Elsevier; 2006. p. 63–73.

20. Coyne MJ. Seroconversion of puppies to canine parvovirus and canine distemper virus: a comparison of two combination vaccines. J Am Anim Hosp Assoc 2000;36(2):137–42.

21. Pratelli A, Cavalli A, Martella V, et al. Canine parvovirus (CPV) vaccination: comparison of neutralizing antibody responses in pups after inoculation with CPV2 or CPV2b modified live virus vaccine. Clin Diagn Lab Immunol 2001;8(3):612–5.

22. Abdelmagid OY, Larson L, Payne L, et al. Evaluation of the efficacy and duration of immunity of a canine combination vaccine against virulent parvovirus, infectious canine hepatitis virus, and distemper virus experimental challenges. Vet Ther 2004;5(3):173–86.

23. Mouzin DE, Lorenzen MJ, Haworth JD, et al. Duration of serologic response to five viral antigens in dogs. J Am Vet Med Assoc 2004;224(1):55–60.

24. National Association of State Public Health Veterinarians. Compendium of animal rabies prevention and control, 2011. J Am Vet Med Assoc 2011;239(5):609–17.

25. Ward MP, Glickman LT, Guptill LF. Prevalence of and risk factors for leptospirosis among dogs in the United States and Canada: 677 cases (1970-1998). J Am Vet Med Assoc 2002;220(1):53–8.

26. Langston CE, Heuter KJ. Leptospirosis: a re-emerging zoonotic disease. Vet Clin North Am Small Anim Pract 2003;33(4):791–807.

27. Ford RB. Companion animal vaccines. In: Ettinger SJ, Feldman EC, editors. Textbook of veterinary internal medicine, vol. 1, 7th edition. St Louis (MO): Elsevier Saunders; 2010. p. 853 Chapter 197.

28. Greene CE, Straubinger RK. Borreliosis. In: Greene CE, editor. Infectious diseases of the dog and cat. 3rd edition. St Louis (MO): Saunders Elsevier; 2006. p. 417–35.

29. Littman MP. Canine borreliosis. Vet Clin North Am Small Anim Pract 2003;33(4): 827–62.

30. Goldstein RE. Lyme disease. In: Ettinger SJ, Feldman EC, editors. Textbook of veterinary internal medicine, vol. 1, 7th edition. St Louis (MO): Elsevier Saunders; 2010. p. 868 Chapter 199.

31. Greene CE, Appel MJ. Canine distemper. In: Greene CE, editor. Infectious diseases of the dog and cat. 3rd edition. St Louis (MO): Saunders Elsevier; 2006. p. 25–41.
32. Pardo MC, Bauman JE, Mackowiak M. Protection of dogs against canine distemper by vaccination with a canarypox virus recombinant expressing canine distemper virus fusion and hemagglutinin glycoproteins. Am J Vet Res 1997; 58(8):833–6.
33. Larson LJ, Henningson J, Sharp P, et al. Efficacy of the canine influenza virus H3N8 vaccine to decrease severity of clinical disease after cochallenge with canine influenza virus and *Streptococcus equi* subsp. *Zooepidemicus*. Clin Vaccine Immunol 2011;18(4):559–64. http://dx.doi.org/10.1128/CVI.00500-10.
34. Wallis DM, Wallis JL. Rattlesnake vaccine to prevent envenomation toxicity in dogs. Presented at the Dr Ross O. Mosier 77th Annual Western Veterinary Conference. Las Vegas (NV), February 20th-24th, 2005.
35. Lappin MJ, Andrews J, Simpson D, et al. Use of serologic tests to predict resistance to feline herpesvirus 1, feline calicivirus, and feline parvovirus infection in cats. J Am Vet Med Assoc 2002;220(1):38–42.
36. Gaskell RM, Dawson S, Radford A. Other feline viral diseases. In: Ettinger SJ, Feldman EC, editors. Textbook of veterinary internal medicine, vol. 1, 7th edition. St Louis (MO): Elsevier Saunders; 2010. p. 946 Chapter 14.
37. Gaskell RM, Dawson S, Radford A. Feline respiratory disease. In: Greene CE, editor. Infectious diseases of the dog and cat. 3rd edition. St Louis (MO): Saunders Elsevier; 2006. p. 145–54.
38. Hurley KF, Sykes JE. Update on feline calicivirus: new trends. Vet Clin North Am Small Anim Pract 2003;33(4):759–72.
39. Hurley KF, Pesavento PA, Pedersen NC, et al. An outbreak of virulent systemic feline calicivirus disease. J Am Vet Med Assoc 2004;224(2):241–9.
40. Krebs JW, Mandel EJ, Swerdlow DL, et al. Rabies Surveillance in the United States during 2003. J Am Vet Med Assoc 2004;225(12):1837–49.
41. Kass PH, Barnes WG, Spangler WL, et al. Epidemiologic evidence for a causal relation between vaccination and fibrosarcoma tumorigenesis in cats. J Am Vet Med Assoc 1993;203(3):396–405.
42. Levy JK, Crawford PC. Feline leukemia virus. In: Ettinger SJ, Feldman EC, editors. Textbook of veterinary internal medicine, vol. 1, 7th edition. St Louis (MO): Elsevier Saunders; 2010. p. 935 Chapter 212.
43. Levy J, Crawford C, Hartmann K, et al. 2008 American Association of Feline Practitioners' feline retrovirus management guidelines. J Feline Med Surg 2008;10(3): 300–16.
44. Greene CE. Chlamydial infections. In: Greene CE, editor. Infectious diseases of the dog and cat. 3rd edition. St Louis (MO): Saunders Elsevier; 2006. p. 245–52.
45. Levy JK, Crawford PC. Feline immunodeficiency virus infection. In: Ettinger SJ, Feldman EC, editors. Textbook of veterinary internal medicine, vol. 1, 7th edition. St Louis (MO): Elsevier Saunders; 2010. p. 929 Chapter 211.
46. Sellon RK, Hartmann K. Feline immunodeficiency virus infection. In: Greene CE, editor. Infectious diseases of the dog and cat. 3rd edition. St Louis (MO): Saunders Elsevier; 2006. p. 131–43.
47. Addie D, Jarrett O. Feline coronavirus infections. In: Greene CE, editor. Infectious diseases of the dog and cat. 3rd edition. St Louis (MO): Saunders Elsevier; 2006. p. 88–102.
48. Hartmann K. Feline infectious peritonitis and feline coronavirus infection. In: Ettinger SJ, Feldman EC, editors. Textbook of veterinary internal medicine, vol. 1, 7th edition. St Louis (MO): Elsevier Saunders; 2010. p. 940.

49. Morrison WB, Starr RM, Vaccine-Associated Feline Sarcoma Task Force. Vaccine-associated feline sarcomas. J Am Vet Med Assoc 2001;218(5):697–702.
50. Vaccine-Associated Feline Sarcoma Task Force. The current understanding and management of vaccine-associated sarcomas in cats. J Am Vet Med Assoc 2005;226(11):1821–42.
51. Tizard I. Resistance to tumors. In: Veterinary immunology. 9th edition. St Louis (MO): Elsevier-Saunders; 2013. p. 387–99.
52. Srivastav A, Kass PH, McGill LD, et al. Comparative vaccine-specific and other injectable-specific risks of injection-site sarcomas in cats. J Am Vet Med Assoc 2012;241(5):595–602.
53. Meyer KE. Vaccine-associated adverse events. Vet Clin North Am Small Anim Pract 2001;31(3):493–514.
54. Tizard I. Immune complexes and type III hypersensitivity. In: Veterinary immunology. 9th edition. St Louis (MO): Elsevier-Saunders; 2013. p. 355–64.

Pediatric Nutrition

Deborah S. Greco, DVM, PhD

KEYWORDS

- Bitch • Puppy • Queen • Kitten • Milk replacer • Probiotics • Prebiotics

KEY POINTS

- Feeding a balanced commercial diet to lactating and growing puppies and kittens provides the necessary macronutrients (protein, fat, and so forth), vitamins, minerals, and supplements required for normal growth and development.
- The most important immune-related function of good intestinal microflora is protection against infection and colonization by harmful, and sometimes pathogenic, bacteria.
- Added benefit may arise from the use of docosahexaenoic acid–supplemented diets and from the use of prebiotic fibers, colostrum, and probiotics to promote growth and development of a healthy gastrointestinal tract, microbiota, and immune system in puppies and kittens.

INTRODUCTION

Balanced commercial dog foods designed for all life stages are the mainstay of feeding for optimal reproductive capacity in the bitch and ideal growth rates in puppies and kittens. Recent evidence suggests that certain micronutrients and macronutrients, when balanced with other nutrients in the formulation, may provide a healthier immune system, balanced gastrointestinal (GI) microbiota, and more acute hearing and vision.

PREGNANT AND LACTATING BITCHES

In general, pregnant and lactating bitches should be fed a high-energy (30% protein; 20% fat on a dry matter basis [DMB]), highly digestible commercial dog food that is balanced for vitamins and minerals. The food should be labeled adequate for all life stages. Food intake should not increase during the first 5 weeks of gestation; however, the food intake requirements increase to 1.25 to 1.5 times maintenance during the last trimester. During pregnancy in the bitch, protein requirements increase by up to 70% compare with maintenance to reach 6.3 g of protein per 419 kJ (100 kcal).[1] High-quality, animal-based proteins are preferred. Protein deficiency during pregnancy can result in low birth weights and high neonatal mortality.[2] During lactation,

Nestle Purina PetCare, One Checkerboard Square, St. Louis, MO 63164, USA
E-mail address: deborah.greco@rdmo.nestle.com

Vet Clin Small Anim 44 (2014) 265–273
http://dx.doi.org/10.1016/j.cvsm.2013.11.001
0195-5616/14/$ – see front matter © 2014 Elsevier Inc. All rights reserved.

protein requirements are even higher, particularly in large litters.[3] Feeding multiple times a day, with concentrated high-quality food, is essential to maintain body condition of the bitch, otherwise milk production decreases and neonatal growth is affected. In queens, certain amino acids such as taurine play an important role in maintenance of pregnancy. Fat delivers more kilojoules per gram of food (twice as many) than carbohydrates or protein, making it an essential component of an energy-rich diet for late gestation and lactation. However, lactation is extremely demanding and energy requirements may increase by 3 times compared with basal requirements by the time of weaning, particularly in large litters. Although protein and fat intake should increase in pregnant and lactating bitches, maintenance of ideal body condition is an important aspect of feeding pregnant and lactating bitches. Bitches that become overweight have a greater chance of pseudocyesis and dystocia.[4]

Before birth, some important nutritional requirements can affect the long-term health and well-being of puppies. Fats and essential fatty acids, such as linoleic and alpha-linoleic acid, are in increased demand during pregnancy and lactation in the bitch. Essential fatty acid deficiency has been associated with preterm labor, poor placental development and small litter size.[1] In particular, dams fed a diet rich in docosahexaenoic acid (DHA) deliver puppies that have improved learning ability, memory, and vision.[5–7]

Pregnant and lactating bitches do not require calcium supplementation unless to balance a homemade diet or to treat eclampsia, if present. The proper calcium/phosphorus ratio in diets for pregnant and lactating bitches is 1:0.8. Normal dietary calcium during gestation does not increase the risk for eclampsia in dogs; oversupplementation can induce parathyroid gland atrophy and associated postpartum hypocalcemia.[1] Concerns have been raised about the role of calcium in the periparturient period. Increased stillbirths have been associated with lower ionized Ca and higher parathyroid hormone levels in German shepherd bitches.[8] During lactation in the bitch, the demand for calcium increases exponentially.[9,10] In particular, small breed dogs such as Chihuahuas may be at increased risk for eclampsia, particularly if they are being fed homemade diets, such as chicken and rice, without calcium supplementation.

Prenatal folate supplementation has been promoted in human medicine to alleviate midline closure defects such as spina bifida and cleft palate. The only study in dogs showed that supplementation of folate in Boston terriers resulted in a decrease in the percentage of puppies with cleft palates.[11] However, the study was performed with dogs fed a homemade diet deficient in grains that contain large amounts of folate.[11]

Prebiotics

Sterile at birth, the GI tract is colonized within hours of birth. This well-controlled colonization involves a variety of organisms that find their own niches along the GI tract so that different groups of microorganisms colonize various locations of the intestinal tract. During the colonization process, these bacteria are organized into a state of equilibrium (a balance between beneficial and harmful bacteria) so that the health of the animal is maintained. In the stomach, because of its oxygen content and acidity, resident bacteria numbers are limited to 10^3 to 10^4 bacteria per gram of stomach contents. The primary bacteria populating the stomach are lactobacilli and enterococci. Bacteria in the small intestine are a combination of facultative anaerobes and anaerobes whose growth is limited by peristaltic activity. Populations of these microorganisms are low in the upper small intestine, but increase throughout the tract from the duodenum to the ileum. The greatest colonization of the GI tract (approximately 200 species or 400 different strains of bacteria) occurs in the colon, where decreased intestinal transit time allows bacteria to reach numbers of 10^{11} to 10^{12} organisms per gram. Bacterial flora in the colon is dominated by anaerobes such as intestinal microflora (*Bacteroides, Eubacterium, Bifidobacterium, Lactobacillus*, and *Enterococcus*).

Because the gut microbiota can play a major role in the health of the host animal, there is significant interest in the manipulation of it toward a potentially more remedial community. Indigestible oligosaccharides, in general, are prebiotic fibers and have been shown to modulate the colonic microbiota by increasing the number of so-called good bacteria, thus changing the composition of the microbiota. The characteristics of a beneficial prebiotic are that it passes unchanged through the digestive system until it reaches the large intestine; it has metabolic selectivity for good bacteria; it alters microflora balance in favor of a healthier composition; and it induces effects that are beneficial to the animal.

Prebiotic fibers have been reported to have benefits such as immune stimulation, anticancer effects, antidiarrhea effects, and increased nutrient absorption. Popular prebiotics include inulin, aleurone, fructo-oligosaccharides (FOSs), mono-oligosaccharides, and beet pulp. Studies have shown that dietary supplementation of short chain fructo oligosaccharides (scFOS) to pregnant and lactating bitches increased colostrum and milk immunoglobulin (Ig) M content without a concomitant effect on IgG1, IgG2, and IgA.[2] Furthermore, intranasally immunized puppies showed higher *Bordetella bronchiseptica*–specific IgM response.[12]

PEDIATRIC PUPPIES: WEANING TO 6 MONTHS

Growth rates differ greatly between small and medium, large, and even giant breed puppies. For example, a miniature poodle may be sexually and physiologically mature at 6 to 8 months of age, whereas a Great Dane may not achieve maturity until 28 to 36 months (3 years) of age. As a result of these breed size differences in the rate of growth, food companies have designed foods for small, medium, large, and giant breeds. The smaller puppy diets are higher in energy and protein, whereas the large and giant breed diets are lower in caloric content but still high enough in protein to allow proper growth and development. Overfeeding large breed puppies has been shown to increase the incidence of osteoarthritis (OA) and obesity.[13] Mismatch in the amount of protein and energy in the diet may result in relative protein deficiency that can cause immune problems and carbohydrate intolerance later in life.[14] Puppy foods that match the amount of protein to the amount of energy in the diet provide the ideal diet for growth in small, large, and giant breed puppies. Ideal foods for growing puppies contain at least 25% protein on a percent energy basis. Feeding instructions should be considered to be guidelines because individual puppies are different and may require adjustments to keep them in a lean body condition (4–5 out of 9 on the Purina scale). Excess body weight is recognized as a risk factor for OA in both humans and dogs, whereas avoiding obesity can help reduce OA. Dogs maintained in lean body condition through food restriction experienced decreased severity, and delayed onset, of OA.[13–16]

The amounts of omega-3 and omega-6 fatty acids are essential to promoting a healthy immune system, skin, and hair coat both in utero and in developing puppies. Foods should contain the proper amount (0.05% DHA, Association of American Feed Control Officials [AAFCO] recommendation) of essential fatty acids, including linoleic acid, for growth and development. Feeding diets rich in DHA to puppies up to 12 weeks in age improves memory and vision. Omega-3 fatty acids, such as DHA, are required for normal development of retinal function and hearing in puppies.

Differences in mineral requirements between large and small breed puppies may be one of the most important aspects of puppy nutrition. Although miniature poodle puppies grow and develop normally on a wide range of calcium intakes, Great Dane puppies require a specific amount (1.5%) of calcium for normal skeletal growth. Skeletal defects (hip dysplasia, panosteitis, and so forth) and depressed growth were observed when high levels of calcium were fed to Great Dane puppies; normal growth and development were observed when the puppies were fed 0.80% to 1.5 % Ca on a DMB.[17] Severely reduced growth and pathologic fractures were noted in Great Dane puppies fed less than or equal to 0.55% Ca on a DMB (low calcium).[17] Small, large, and giant breed puppy foods have varying amounts of calcium and phosphorus in the proper ratios to control growth and development of bones and cartilage. The adult size of a puppy is not determined by the rate of growth (accelerated beyond normal), but by the genetic makeup of the puppy (the size of the parents). Again, slower, more controlled growth of the skeleton is associated with more normal development. Rapid growth has been associated with the development of OA, osteochondrosis dissecans, hip dysplasia, and metabolic bone disease in large and giant breed dogs.[15,17] Calcium supplements should not be used because of the detrimental effects on bone growth, particularly in large breed puppies. Natural supplements, such as yogurt and cottage cheese, contain excessive amounts of calcium; for example, yogurt contains 450 mg of Ca per cup.

SUPPLEMENTS THAT AFFECT THE IMMUNE SYSTEM IN PUPPIES AND KITTENS

The gut is the largest immune system organ in the body. About 70% of the body's immune system is located in the GI tract. As such, the interaction between the gut-associated lymphoid tissue and microflora is key to overall health. The most important immune-related function of the good intestinal microflora is protection against infection and colonization by harmful, and sometimes pathogenic, bacteria. This protection is provided by physical barriers and resistance to pathogen colonization. Both of these protective mechanisms can be altered by several factors. Aging and stress associated with traveling, kennel boarding, changes in environment or diet, and poor nutrition also can affect the balance. One study that investigated the effects of aging on the intestinal microflora of dogs found that young adult dogs had higher levels of lactobacilli and lower levels of Clostridium perfringens compared with elderly dogs.[1] Stress can trigger changes in intestinal pH, contractility, and transit time, resulting in an imbalance in microflora. Shifts in microbial populations can result in increased shedding of pathogenic bacteria and reduced performance of the protective barrier of the gut, which can lead to GI upset and systemic problems. Even otherwise good stresses, such as traveling for a competitive dog event, can upset this delicate balance. Two recent advances in veterinary nutrition, bovine colostrum supplementation and probiotic therapy, may help prevent some of the digestive upset associated with unavoidable stressors such as weaning and travel.

Colostrum

As nutritional science has become more advanced, certain nutrients and ingredients have been identified that provide more benefit to the animal than was previously thought. Colostrum is one of these entities that provides more benefit than was previously thought. Neonatal mammals acquire passive immunity during the first 24 hours of life because a permeable GI tract allows large immunoglobulins in the first mother's milk to pass freely through the intestinal barrier for about 24 to 48 hours after birth. However, it seems that kittens and puppies may have a shorter window for transfer of factors, with optimum transfer in the first 3 to 6 hours and completion by 16 to 24 hours.[18,19] These nutrients and ingredients contain bioactive compounds that positively influence both the immune and GI systems. Bovine colostrum has been identified as one such immunostimulatory bioactive ingredient. Recent research has shown that natural antibodies (also called immunoglobulins) and other bioactive growth factors found in colostrum can help strengthen the immature immune system of a puppy or kitten. It can help balance the beneficial and harmful bacteria in the intestine, which not only promotes nutrient absorption facilitated by colonic microflora but lowers the potential for infection, diarrhea, and intestinal inflammation. In addition, it is a good source of readily available amino acids for gut cell health and barrier function.

Although the neonate is born with a functional immune system, it is still immature and naive at birth. Its response to any immunostimulation is that of a first exposure, requiring a prolonged period to produce immunoglobulins. Colostrum provides immunoglobulins and other bioactive growth factors that stimulate development of the GI tract.

The importance of colostrum in helping establish a healthy intestinal microflora population has been investigated.[20-22] Human studies show that breastfed infants have a predominance of beneficial bacteria (bifidobacteria and lactobacilli) and lower fecal pH compared with those fed a pasteurized cow milk–based formulation. The endogenous intestinal bacteria compete with pathogens and provide an environment that favors beneficial bacteria. In addition to the physical barrier provided by the mucous membranes lining the GI tract and the immunologic power of gut-associated lymphoid tissue, the intestinal microflora have an important role as part of the body's natural defense system.

New research has been conducted to investigate the use of colostrum to enhance immunity and modulate gut microflora in both kittens and puppies.[22] Colostrum is a combination of secretions from the mammary gland and proteins transferred from the blood stream. Many studies suggest that various constituents of milk are bioactive because of their positive health effects. For example, bovine milk components represent a potentially useful way to modulate gut microflora and immunity. Bovine colostrum and the whey fraction (a protein-rich complex derived from bovine milk) contain not only immunoglobulins but also lactoferrin, lactoglobulin, lactalbumin, all of which have been shown to modulate immune function as well as intestinal microflora. Lactoferrin inhibits undesirable microflora by sequestering iron in the gut, and promotes the growth of the beneficial bacteria, lactobacilli and bifidobacteria. Glycomacropeptide is known to regulate appetite as well as act as a prebiotic and immunostimulant. Cytokines and growth factors such as epidermal growth factor, tumor growth factor alpha, tumor growth factor R, insulinlike growth factors and binding proteins, platelet-derived growth factor, vascular endothelial growth factor, and growth hormone play important roles in maintaining a healthy gut wall.

Immunoglobulins are Y-shaped molecules in which the shorter arm of the Y is named the fragment antigen binding (Fab) region and the longer body is named the fragment crystalline (Fc) region. The Fab region binds specific antigens, whereas the Fc region is responsible for most of the biologic activity by interacting with the immune cells. Most of the immunoglobulins introduced into the gut remain intact through the stomach into the small intestine where the immune cells reside. Slight denaturing may enhance the ability of the Fc region to bind immune cells and stimulate the immune system. When colostrum is delivered with a complete and balanced diet there is ample food matrix available for degradation by the stomach enzymes, which in turn causes decreased pH. Immunoglobulins are small and therefore not a high priority for processing by the stomach before entering the small intestines. Based on studies in other species, the relevant components of the immunoglobulins remain intact through digestion and have a positive immunomodulating effect on digestion. As a result, most immunoglobulins in the diet reach the small intestine, where they bind and stimulate immune cells and boost the immune status of the animal. Therefore, the ultimate benefits of immunoglobulins are their ability to bind the gut immune cells, which in turn stimulates the local and systemic immune system and results in overall enhanced immunity.

One of the protective functions of the gut is to eliminate pathogenic bacteria and neutralize toxins. Bioactives in colostrum have been shown to bind specific receptors on the gut immune cells and activate them to secrete higher levels of IgA into the lumen of the gut. Secretory IgA prevents adherence of pathogens to mucosal surfaces, transports potential pathogens out of the cells into the lumen, binds virus, and prevents replication. The gut IgA is eventually excreted in the feces. Therefore, a higher level of fecal IgA is desirable because it indicates stimulation of the local mucosal immune system. Colostrum stimulates the gut immune system to secrete higher levels of secretory IgA.

Bacterial populations are in constant flux in the gut because of cellular turnover, introduction of food, and interaction of the gut microenvironment. Puppies and kittens fed the colostrum diet had more similarity in their microbial population before and after stress. A more stable microbial population leads to optimized nutrient absorption and decreased susceptibility to stress-induced or stress-related diarrhea.

A complete and balanced diet supplemented with colostrum enhanced the systemic immune status and digestive health of puppies and kittens without causing overstimulation of the immune system. In addition, the puppies and kittens fed colostrum had higher fecal IgA, indicating a higher local gut immune response. Increased similarity of bacterial populations in the gut before and after stress, natural antibodies, and other bioactives in colostrum help to balance beneficial and potentially harmful intestinal bacteria. By stabilizing gut microflora, colostrum helps promote nutrient absorption and lowers the potential for infection, diarrhea, and intestinal inflammation.

Probiotics

Enterococci are typical lactic acid bacteria and occur naturally in a wide variety of environments, including certain foods, as well as in the intestinal tract of animals. Much human research has been conducted on the potential benefits of SF68 in patients with acute diarrhea, traveler's diarrhea, dysbiosis associated with antibiotic use, irritable bowel syndrome, hepatic disorders, and encephalopathy. Probiotics have been shown to decrease the incidence, severity, and duration of diarrhea.

In selecting a potential strain to be used as a probiotic for a pet food supplement, several important factors should be considered, including a long history of safe use in both humans and animals, and whether it has been approved by AAFCO. The potential benefits of SF68, based on a large number of trials in humans and animals, were consistent with desirable benefits in pets. Probiotics have been shown to survive the conditions of the GI tract in pets based on well-controlled in vitro and in vivo tests. Certain probiotics (such as FortiFlora; Nestle Purina, Vevey, Switzerland) incorporate a proprietary microencapsulation process that allow for stability of the microorganisms through the production, distribution, and storage processes.

Probiotics have been used successfully in both dogs and cats since 1985 for the maintenance and restoration of healthy gut microflora in animals showing disturbances caused by changes in diet, stress, and antibiotic therapy. *Enterococcus faecium* can temporarily survive in the GI tract of healthy adult dogs for about 14 days. Feeding *E faecium* reduced the fecal concentration of *C perfringens* in dogs and increased levels of fecal bifidobacteria and lactobacilli. Probiotics caused statistically significant improvement in fecal scores in dogs with naturally occurring diarrhea.[23]

Puppies and kittens can be susceptible to diarrhea, particularly at the time of weaning or if insufficient colostrum has been ingested. In both cases, administration of probiotics, like E faecium, repopulates the intestine with helpful bacteria for 14 days to allow repair and stabilization of gut flora. Other probiotics are available from several different pharmaceutical companies; however, most of them have not undergone rigorous clinical trials and studies to prove efficacy. Yogurt contains too much calcium to be used as a probiotic and most yogurts do not contain sufficient measurable amounts of beneficial bacteria to be considered probiotics. The manufacturer should be able to provide documentation as to whether the probiotic has stability (ie, it does not revert to a pathogenic strain), and whether it survives in the gut for a least 14 days.

The microflora in the GI tract consists of normal and pathogenic microflora. The helpful microorganisms contribute to intestinal mucosal integrity, metabolism, and immune status (both local and systemic). In addition, probiotics or live active cultures have been shown to have beneficial effects in the host animal by improving its intestinal microbial balance. However, one of the most interesting studies on the effects of E faecium found that there were statistically significant increases in IgA observed in animals fed the probiotic.[22] In cats, decreased recurrence of clinical signs of herpes virus during stress was also observed when the cats were supplemented with probiotics.[23] This boosting of the immune system in puppies and kittens has important implications for improving the health of pets and the immune response to vaccination.

MILK REPLACERS FOR ORPHANED PUPPIES AND KITTENS

The composition of bitch and queen milk compared with commercially available milk replacers is shown in **Table 1**. Although there is not much literature pertaining to milk replacement therapy in orphaned puppies and kittens, a few studies could be found.[24,25] The use of a commercially available puppy milk replacer in Denmark was associated with overfeeding of puppies; furthermore, the milk replacer had 7-fold the recommend content of vitamin D.[24] The investigators concluded that this could result in abnormal skeletal growth and developmental orthopedic problems later in life. There were similar findings of increased weight gain in kittens fed a commercial milk replacer (CMR) compared with kittens fed queen's milk.[25] In addition, kittens fed the CMR had diarrhea through most of the trial period and most of them developed diffuse anterior and posterior lens opacification.[25] Serum arginine was significantly

Table 1
Comparison of the macronutrient content (percent dry matter [DM]) of commercial milk replacers to species-specific milk composition

Type	Protein (% DM)	Fat (% DM)	Carbohydrates (% DM)
Bitch milk	33	41	17
Queen milk	42	25	26
Commercial goat milk (Esbilac)	35	42	15
Veterinary dog (Nutri-Cal[a])	34	43	16
Commercial dog (Just Born[b])	30	30	30
Commercial cat (KMR)	44	26	24

[a] Contains FOS, colostrums.
[b] Contains colostrum, and arginine to prevent cataracts.

lower in the CMR-fed kittens and may have contributed to the cataract formation. Based on these findings, currently available milk replacers are often supplemented with arginine and more restricted in vitamin D supplementation than previously available preparations. Clients should be instructed to follow manufacturer's feeding instructions carefully and not to overfeed.

SUMMARY

Feeding a balanced commercial diet to lactating and growing puppies and kittens provides the necessary macronutrients (protein, fat, and so forth), vitamins, minerals, and supplements required for normal growth and development. Added benefit may arise from the use of DHA-supplemented diets and from the use of prebiotic fibers, colostrum, and probiotics to promote growth and development of a healthy GI tract, microbiota, and immune system in puppies and kittens.

REFERENCES

1. Kirk CA. New concepts in pediatric nutrition [review]. Vet Clin North Am Small Anim Pract 2001;31(2):369–92.
2. Ontko JA, Phillips PH. Reproduction and lactation studies with bitches fed semi-purified diets. J Nutr 1958;65:211–8.
3. Schroeder GE, Smith GA. Bodyweight and feed intake of German shepherd bitches during pregnancy and lactation. J Small Anim Pract 1995;36(1):7–11.
4. Lawler DF, Johnston SD, Keltner DG, et al. Influence of restricted food intake on estrous cycles and pseudopregnancies in dogs. Am J Vet Res 1999; 60(7):820–5.
5. Heinemann KM, Waldron MK, Bigley KE, et al. Long-chain (n-3) polyunsaturated fatty acids are more efficient than alpha-linolenic acid in improving electroretinogram responses of puppies exposed during gestation, lactation, and weaning. J Nutr 2005;135(8):1960–6.
6. Heinemann KM, Bauer JE. Docosahexaenoic acid and neurologic development in animals [review]. J Am Vet Med Assoc 2006;228(5):700–5, 655.
7. Bauer JE, Heinemann KM, Bigley KE, et al. Maternal diet alpha-linolenic acid during gestation and lactation does not increase docosahexaenoic acid in canine milk. J Nutr 2004;134(Suppl 8):2035S–8S.
8. Hollingshead. Calcium and parathormone concentrations in German shepherd bitches during labor (abstract). Proc World Sm Anim Vet Asso. 2007.
9. Adkins Y, Lepine AJ, Lönnerdal B. Changes in protein and nutrient composition of milk throughout lactation in dogs. Am J Vet Res 2001;62(8):1266–72.
10. Lawler DF. The role of perinatal care in development [review]. Semin Vet Med Surg (Small Anim) 1995;10(1):59–67.
11. Elwood JM, Colquhoun TA. Observations on the prevention of cleft palate in dogs by folic acid and the potential relevance to humans. N Z Vet J 1997;45(6):254–6.
12. Adogony V, Respondek F, Biourge V, et al. Effects of dietary scFOS on immunoglobulins in colostrum and milk of bitches. J Anim Physiol Anim Nutr (Berl) 2007; 91:169–74.
13. Dobenecker B, Endres V, Kienzle E. Energy requirements of puppies of two different breeds for ideal growth from weaning to 28 weeks of age. J Anim Physiol Anim Nutr (Berl) 2013;97:190–6.
14. Kealy RD, Lawler DF, Ballam JM, et al. Effects of diet restriction on life span and age-related changes in dogs. J Am Vet Med Assoc 2002;220(9):1315–20.

15. Nap RC, Hazewinkel HA, Voorhout G, et al. Growth and skeletal development in Great Dane pups fed different levels of protein intake. J Nutr 1991;121(Suppl 11): S107–13.
16. Kealy RD, Lawler DF, Ballam JM, et al. Evaluation of the effect of limited food consumption on radiographic evidence of osteoarthritis in dogs. J Am Vet Med Assoc 2000;217(11):1678–80.
17. Schoenmakers I, Hazewinkel HA, Voorhout G, et al. Effects of diets with different calcium and phosphorus contents on the skeletal development of growing Great Danes. Vet Rec 2000;147(23):652–60.
18. Chastant-Maillard S, Freyburger L, Marcheteau E, et al. Timing of the intestinal barrier closure in puppies. Reprod Domest Anim 2012;47(Suppl 6):190–3.
19. Casal ML, Jezyk PF, Giger U. Transfer of colostral antibodies from queens to their kittens. Am J Vet Res 1996;57(11):1653–8.
20. Giffard CJ, Seino MM, Markwell PJ, et al. Benefits of bovine colostrum on fecal quality in recently weaned puppies. J Nutr 2004;134:2126S–7S.
21. Satyaraj E, Reynolds A, Pelker R, et al. Supplementation of diets with bovine colostrum influences immune function in dogs. Br J Nutr 2013;1–6.
22. Benyacoub J, Czarnecki-Maulden GL, Cavadini C, et al. Supplementation of food with *Enterococcus faecium* (SF68) stimulates immune functions in young dogs. J Nutr 2003;133(4):1158–62.
23. Lappin MR, Veir JK, Satyaraj E, et al. Pilot study to evaluate the effect of oral supplementation of *Enterococcus faecium* SF68 on cats with latent feline herpes virus 1. J Feline Med Surg 2009;11:650.
24. Corbee RJ, Tryfonidou MA, Beckers IP, et al. Composition and use of puppy milk replacers in German Shepherd puppies in the Netherlands. J Anim Physiol Anim Nutr (Berl) 2012;96:395–402.
25. Remillard RL, Pickett JP, Thatcher CD, et al. Comparison of kittens fed queen's milk with those fed milk replacers. Am J Vet Res 1993;54:901–7.

Pediatric Seizure Disorders in Dogs and Cats

James A. Lavely, DVM

KEYWORDS

- Pediatric neurology • Dog • Cat • Seizures • Distemper • *Neospora* • *Cryptococcus*

KEY POINTS

- Seizure disorders in young animals pose different considerations as to cause and therapeutic decisions compared with adult animals.
- Infectious diseases of the nervous system are more likely in puppies and kittens compared with adults.
- The diagnosis of canine distemper is often based on clinical signs, with the combination of neurologic abnormalities, particularly myoclonus, with extraneural signs leading to a high suspicion of canine distemper in dogs less than 1 year old.
- Idiopathic epilepsy typically occurs in dogs between 1 and 5 years of age; however, inflammatory brain diseases such as necrotizing encephalitis and granulomatous meningoencephalomyelitis also commonly occur in young to middle-aged small-breed dogs.
- The choice of anticonvulsant for maintenance therapy is tailored to each individual patient.

Seizures are the manifestation of abnormal synchronous electrical activity in the brain and are the most common neurologic disorder in dogs. Seizures may be categorized as generalized, when both cerebral hemispheres are involved, or partial, when cerebral involvement is focal. Generalized seizures result in loss of consciousness and the whole body is affected with signs such as paddling, convulsions, or increased tone. Salivation is common and some animals may urinate, defecate, or vomit at the time of the seizure. Partial seizures affect only a portion of the body. Consciousness is unimpaired during simple partial seizures and is altered during complex partial seizures. During psychomotor seizures, a complex partial seizure, the animal may appear panicked as it compulsively runs around, and may appear aggressive, hissing or growling. A preictal period before the seizure and a postictal period lasting minutes to hours after the seizure are common with generalized seizures. Preictal and postictal signs may include anxiety, attention seeking, panting, and pacing. The recognition of seizures can sometimes be difficult because vestibular episodes, dyskinesias, and syncopal episodes can appear seizurelike. A

Department of Neurology and Neurosurgery, VCA Animal Care Center of Sonoma, 6470 Redwood Drive, Rohnert Park, CA 94928, USA
E-mail address: james.lavely@vcahospitals.com

Vet Clin Small Anim 44 (2014) 275–301
http://dx.doi.org/10.1016/j.cvsm.2013.10.004
0195-5616/14/$ – see front matter © 2014 Elsevier Inc. All rights reserved.

thorough history should be gathered including the potential for toxin exposure, familial history, previous events, activity during onset, time of onset, duration of the event, elimination during the event, and interictal behavioral or gait changes. In the pediatric patient, information regarding birth, litter mates, suckling, and weight gain is also important. Seizure disorders in young animals pose different considerations as to cause and therapeutic decisions compared with adult animals. Congenital, developmental, metabolic, toxic, infectious, and inflammatory causes are considered more likely in puppies and kittens.

A thorough evaluation for the underlying cause for seizures should be pursued to optimize anticonvulsant therapy. Patients with underlying causes other than idiopathic epilepsy may require medication in addition to anticonvulsant therapy. In addition, patients with secondary epilepsy often require anticonvulsant therapy sooner than those with primary/idiopathic epilepsy. Complete blood count (CBC), serum chemistry, and urinalysis should be done for all dogs and cats presenting for seizures. Hypoglycemia should be ruled out in all puppies and kittens. Bile acid testing is important in all puppies and small-breed dogs.

PORTOSYSTEMIC SHUNTS

Portosystemic shunts (PSSs) are common in small-breed dogs (Yorkshire terrier, Maltese terrier, and miniature schnauzer) and are commonly diagnosed at less than 2 years of age. Congenital extrahepatic PSSs are usually single vessels that connect the portal venous system to the systemic circulation. They may arise from any vessel and account for most shunts. Portocaval shunts are more common than portoazygous shunts.[1] PSS in large-breed dogs are typically intrahepatic in location. PSS often causes episodic encephalopathic signs such as mentation changes, head pressing, vocalization, ataxia, blindness, and seizures. Between 79% and 82% of dogs have central nervous system (CNS) signs associated with PSS.[1,2] Neurologic signs are typically worse after eating and often wax and wane. Other signs include vomiting, anorexia, polyuria, polydipsia, decreased weight, hematuria, and stranguria. The cause of hepatic encephalopathy is unclear, with several potential causes including hyperammonemia, altered tryptophan synthesis, false neurotransmitter synthesis, alterations in amino acid neurotransmitters, and increased cerebral endogenous benzodiazepine concentrations.[3]

Serum albumin and blood urea nitrogen are typically decreased in dogs with PSS. Preprandial and postprandial bile acids are increased in 95% and 98% of dogs with extrahepatic PSSs. Mean preprandial and postprandial bile acids were 139.9 and 248.2 μmol/L respectively in a study of 168 dogs with single extrahepatic shunts. Ammonium biurate or uric acid crystalluria is common.[1] Hyperammonemia is also a common finding. Mean serum ammonia was 206 μmol/L in dogs and 295 μmol/L in cats with PSS in one study.[4] The sensitivity of increased ammonia was 85% in dogs and 83% in cats. The specificity of ammonia was 86% in dogs and 76% in cats. The sensitivity of increased bile acids was 93% in dogs and 100% in cats. The specificity of bile acids was 67% in dogs and 71% in cats.[4]

Abdominal radiographs typically indicate microhepatica. Confirmation of PSS may be done via abdominal ultrasound or nuclear scintigraphy. The overall sensitivity of ultrasonography was 92% and specificity was 98% in one study. Ultrasonography identified 38 of 42 (90%) extrahepatic PSSs in dogs and cats, and 11 of 11 intrahepatic shunts. Ultrasonography correctly identified the extrahepatic location as portocaval or portoazygous 90% (34 of 38) of the time and correctly identified the location 11 of 11 times in intrahepatic shunts (**Figs. 1** and **2**).[5]

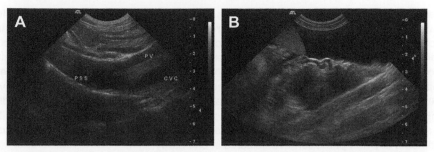

Fig. 1. Abdominal ultrasound. (*A*) Intrahepatic portosystemic shunt. (*B*) Extrahepatic (tortuous) shunt vessel seen lateral to the spleen. Ascites is evident. (*Courtesy of* Tom Baker, MS, Davis, CA.)

Medical therapy for PSS consists of dietary modification, antibiotic therapy, and lactulose with the goal of decreasing NH_3 production. A low-protein diet consisting of high-quality digestible protein is recommended. Commercially available liver disease diets or home-cooked diets with chicken, cottage cheese, rice, and pasta are typically fed. Feeding smaller portions more frequently may be beneficial. Ampicillin 22 mg/kg intravenously (IV) every 6 hours or metronidazole 7.5 to 10 mg/kg by mouth twice a day are commonly used to decrease NH_3-producing bacteria. Lactulose acidifies colonic contents leading to conversion of NH_3 to NH_4. Lactulose also decreases fecal transit time, thereby speeding the elimination of bacteria and NH_3. Lactulose is given to effect, to produce a soft stool. Gastrointestinal ulceration is an increased risk in patients with PSS. Thus, gastric protectants such as famotidine 0.5 mg/kg by mouth twice a day or omeprazole 0.5 to 1 mg/kg by mouth every 24 hours should be given.[6] Anticonvulsant therapy is indicated if seizures are present or given perioperatively.

Surgical ligation/constriction is recommended when possible. Surgery redirects the flow of blood to the hepatic parenchyma. Various techniques are available, including surgical ligation or partial ligation, or the use of devices that gradually occlude the aberrant vessel, such as an ameroid constrictor or a cellophane band. The use of ameroid constrictors and cellophane bands has decreased mortality associated with surgery. Surgical therapy is typically considered superior to medical therapy; however, both therapies can be beneficial. A study comparing surgical therapy with medical therapy indicated a shunt-related mortality of 10.1% of dogs treated surgically versus

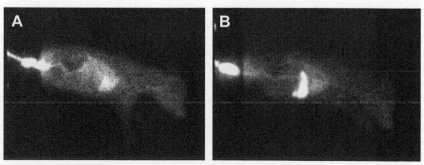

Fig. 2. Nuclear scintigraphy. (*A*) The radioactive material bypasses the liver and is identified in the heart. (*B*) Negative for a shunt after surgical correction. The radioactive material is noted in the liver. (*Courtesy of* Rich Larson, Davis, CA.)

a shunt-related mortality of 29.6% of dogs treated medically. Perioperative mortality was 4% in this study.[7] Postoperative seizures are reported in 5% to 18% of dogs surgically and typically occur within 3 days of surgery.[2,8] Neurologic signs may occur from decreased circulating endogenous benzodiazepine ligands, imbalances in excitatory or inhibitory neurotransmitters,[8] or hypoglycemia.[2] Postoperative generalized seizures have been associated with high mortality, whereas dogs with postoperative partial seizures typically respond to therapy.[1] Although phenobarbital therapy did not significantly reduce the incidence of seizures, it did seem to reduce the severity of seizures in a study.[2] None of 42 dogs treated with levetiracetam 20 mg/kg by mouth 3 times a day had postoperative seizures in one study.[8]

HYDROCEPHALUS

Hydrocephalus is an increase in cerebrospinal fluid (CSF) volume and should be considered in toy and brachiocephalic breeds. A dome-shaped head or persistent fontanelle may be present. Stenosis of the mesencephalic aqueduct is the most common cause of hydrocephalus. The stenosis typically results in fusion of the rostral colliculi.[9] CSF accumulates rostral to the obstruction and cerebral cortical atrophy occurs. Tearing of ependymal cells and periventricular diverticula can occur from dilatation of the ventricular system.[10] Hydrocephalus may also result from neoplasia or infection obstructing CSF flow. Hydrocephalus was reported secondary to a leiomyosarcoma in a 2-month-old Chihuahua.[11] Cats may develop hydrocephalus secondary to infectious causes such as feline infectious peritonitis (FIP). Hydrocephalus can result from autosomal recessive inheritance in Siamese cats.[12]

The degree of clinical signs from hydrocephalus is variable. Most hydrocephalic animals are asymptomatic. Ventriculomegaly is a common incidental finding in toy and brachiocephalic breeds.[13] Clinical signs can result from alterations in intracranial pressure, loss of cortical neurons or neuronal function, or periventricular edema secondary to abnormal CSF flow across ventricular walls. Clinical signs depend on the anatomic location most affected. Cerebral, vestibular, and cerebellar signs can be seen. A ventral and/or lateral strabismus can occur because of a skull or orbit deformity or from increased pressure on the mesencephalic tegmentum (**Fig. 3**).[14] A thinned calvarium, decreased cerebral tissue, and changes in cerebral vascularity can cause hydrocephalic animals to be more sensitive to head trauma. A hemorrhagic event can lead to acute neurologic deterioration. Chronic subdural hematomas have been identified in a hydrocephalic dog.[15]

Diagnosis is made via cranial magnetic resonance imaging (MRI) or CT scan. Ultrasound through a persistent fontanelle may also be used in the diagnosis (**Fig. 4**). CT scan effectively evaluates the ventricular system. However, beam hardening artifact can obscure evaluation of the brainstem. The superior soft tissue imaging of MRI allows the most detailed evaluation of the disorder. MRI provides superior evaluation of the ventricular system and brainstem.[14,16] MRI can help rule out other causes for hydrocephalus such as infection and neoplasia and can evaluate for concurrent hemorrhage (**Fig. 5**). CSF analysis is important to rule out concurrent inflammatory or infectious disorders.

Medical therapy is indicated when hydrocephalus causes clinical signs. Medical therapy is directed at decreasing CSF production and decreasing periventricular edema. Glucocorticoids decrease CSF production by decreasing Na-K-ATPase activity[17] and may be beneficial if periventricular edema is present. Prednisone is started at 0.5 mg/kg by mouth twice a day and is tapered to the lowest effective dose. Omeprazole also decreases CSF production and may be of benefit. The action of

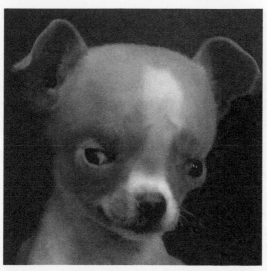

Fig. 3. Chihuahua with hydrocephalus. Note the dome-shaped head and lateral strabismus oculus uterque (OU).

omeprazole action may be independent Na-K-ATPase inhibition.[18] Acetazolamide, a carbonic anhydrase inhibitor, may be of benefit and is given at 10 mg/kg by mouth every 6 to 8 hours. Electrolytes should be monitored with acetazolamide therapy because it can cause hypokalemia.[14,16] Anticonvulsant therapy is indicated when hydrocephalus causes seizures.

Surgical placement of a ventriculoperitoneal shunt is considered for dogs with progressive signs not responsive to medical therapy (**Fig. 6**). Success with shunting is variable. Shunts have not been proved to be more effective than medical therapy. However, shunting does offer the possibility of long-term control of clinical signs.[14] A study of ventriculoperitoneal shunting for congenital hydrocephalus in 36 dogs and cats indicated improved clinical signs in 72% of patients. Complications occurred in 22% of patients, typically within the first 3 months after shunt placement. Median

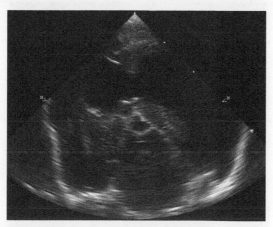

Fig. 4. Transverse ultrasound through a persistent fontanelle at the level of the midbrain. The lateral ventricles are dilated.

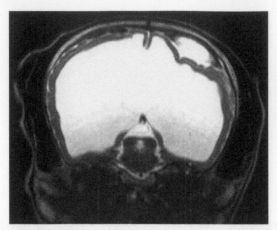

Fig. 5. Transverse T2-weighted MRI. Severe hydrocephalus. An extra-axial hyperintense mass is present. MRI characteristics of the mass indicate a hemorrhage.

follow-up in this study was 6 months, thus complications could be higher. Thirty-six percent of patients died of hydrocephalus-related complications or were euthanized. The 3-month postsurgical survival rate was 66% and the 18-month survival rate was 55%.[19] Two smaller canine studies indicated postoperative complication rates of 25%[20] and 29%.[21]

Potential complications of shunting include infection, occlusion of the shunt, undershunting, overshunting, shunt migration,[19,22] and valve fracture.[21] The need for surgical revision is common in people. Shunt failure occurred in 177 of 344 hydrocephalic children. Only 48% of the shunts were still successful 1 year after shunt implantation. The most common reason for failure was shunt obstruction.[22]

L-2 HYDROXYGLUTARIC ACIDURIA

A metabolic defect causing L-2 hydroxyglutaric aciduria has been recognized in Staffordshire bull terriers,[23] the West Highland white terrier,[24] and the Yorkshire terrier.[25]

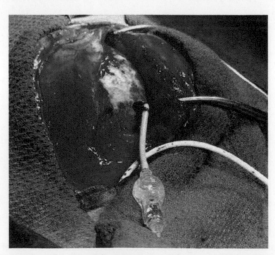

Fig. 6. Surgical placement of a shunt in a coyote with severe hydrocephalus.

L-2 hydroxyglutaric aciduria is an autosomal recessive disease in the Staffordshire bull terrier. The genetic mutation has been identified on exon 10 of chromosome 8 in the Staffordshire bull terrier.[26] This mutation is different than the mutation in the Yorkshire terrier.[25] Clinical signs of L-2 hydroxyglutaric aciduria include seizures, ataxia, stiff gait, decreased mentation, and head tremors. Signs occur from 4 months to 7 years of age, but are often identified at less than 1 year of age. Organic acid analysis of urine, CSF, and plasma are abnormal in affected dogs. MRI identified bilaterally symmetric, diffuse hyperintensity on T2 imaging in the gray matter throughout the brain. No effective treatment is known at this time, other than symptomatic anticonvulsant therapy. Dietary therapy may be of benefit. Cobalamin therapy may be beneficial in methylmalonic aciduria in people.[23] A 6-month-old Cavalier King Charles spaniel was reported to have seizures secondary to a hexanoylglycine aciduria. L-Carnitine therapy is recommended in people with medium-chain acyl coenzyme A dehydrogenase deficiency and thus may be of benefit for hexanoylglycine aciduria.[27]

LISSENCEPHALY

Lissencephaly is a congenital abnormality thought to occur from the arrest of neuronal migration to the cortical plate during fetal development. Lissencephaly results in a smooth cerebral cortical surface as gyri and sulci fail to develop. The cerebral cortex becomes thicker than normal. Fusion of the corpus callosum and internal capsule cause the corona radiata (white matter) to be absent.[9,28] Lissencephaly most commonly is reported in the Lhasa apso.[9,28–30] It has also been reported in the wire-haired fox terrier, the Irish setter and in Korat cats.[9] Seizures are common and may be seen at 1 year of age. Behavioral changes, circling, and visual deficits may also be seen.[9,28,30] Diagnosis is made via MRI (**Fig. 7**). Symptomatic anticonvulsant therapy is recommended.

GRANULOMATOUS MENINGOENCEPHALOMYELITIS

Granulomatous meningoencephalomyelitis (GME) accounts for 5% to 25% of all CNS disorders in dogs. Young to middle-aged small-breed dogs are most commonly affected. However, any age or breed may develop GME. On histology, GME is

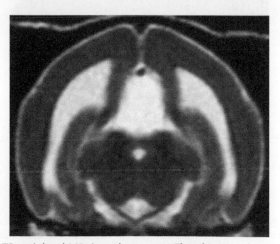

Fig. 7. Transverse T2-weighted MRI in a Lhasa apso. The absence of gyri and sulci indicates lissencephaly. (*Courtesy of* Gregg Kortz, DVM, Sacramento, CA.)

characterized by perivascular cuffs of primarily mononuclear cells within white matter. The accumulation of inflammatory cells is typically microscopic, but areas can coalesce to form a focal granulomatous mass. On histology, the brainstem is commonly involved. Multifocal disease is common, and all regions of the CNS (cerebrum, cerebellum, brainstem, and cervical spinal cord) may be affected. Ocular GME has also been reported. Clinical signs vary based on the region of the CNS involved. The onset may be acute or chronic.[31]

The cause of GME remains unclear. A T cell–mediated delayed-type hypersensitivity reaction with an autoimmune basis is suspected. Infectious causes have been explored and have not been identified. The combination of a nonspecific immunologic response and genetic and environmental factors are all considered likely to play roles in the cause of GME.[32]

Definitive diagnosis of GME can only be made via histopathology. However, a presumptive diagnosis is made antemortem, in the absence of brain biopsy, via a combination of MRI and CSF results. CBC, serum chemistry, and urinalysis are unremarkable. CSF is the single most useful test in inflammatory brain disease.[33] CSF typically yields a mononuclear pleocytosis with increased protein; however, a mixed pleocytosis with an increased percentage of neutrophils is common. CSF results in GME can sometimes mimic the results of other inflammatory brain diseases. Brain imaging can be helpful in differentiating GME from other inflammatory brain disease such as necrotizing meningoencephalitis (NME) and necrotizing leukoencephalitis (NLE). NME and NLE have characteristic abnormalities on MRI that, if present, can help differentiate them from GME. In GME, MRI results often identify edema (hyperintense lesions on T2 and fluid-attenuated inversion recovery [FLAIR]) and contrast-enhancing lesions (**Fig. 8**). MRI abnormalities are typically located within white matter consistent with the histologic distribution of the disease. At times, patients with GME have normal MRI results.[34]

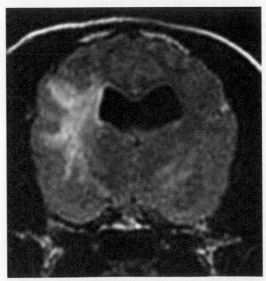

Fig. 8. Transverse FLAIR MRI in a cockapoo. Note the significant hyperintense lesion in the white matter and a smaller hyperintense lesion in the opposite thalamus. CSF indicated a white blood cell count (WBC) of 668 cells/μL and a protein of 462 mg/dL. MRI and CSF findings are consistent with GME.

The mainstay of treatment is corticosteroids. Prednisone is used to treat CNS edema as well as to suppress the immune system. In rapidly deteriorating dogs or in dysphagic dogs, dexamethasone sodium phosphate 0.25 mg/kg IV or subcutaneously every 24 hours to twice a day is given. Prednisone at 1 mg/kg by mouth twice a day is later given. In severe or refractory cases, cytosine arabinoside may be given at 50 mg/m² twice a day for 2 consecutive days and then repeated if necessary every 3 weeks. As an alternative, procarbazine at 25 mg/m² by mouth every 24 hours[35] or cyclosporine 3 to 15 mg/kg by mouth twice a day[36] may be given. Routine monitoring of the CBC should be done when these drugs are given. Serial urinalysis with or without culture is also recommended in immunosuppressed dogs. Clinical signs and serial CSF evaluation are used to assess therapeutic success. Prednisone is tapered over a period of several months. Many dogs require long-term prednisone therapy. Adjunctive therapy such as cytosine arabinoside, cyclosporine, or procarbazine may lessen the dependence on corticosteroids and lead to a more favorable prognosis. The prognosis for GME has been considered guarded. The median survival time for dogs with focal signs was 114 days, whereas dogs with multifocal signs had a median survival time of 8 days in one study.[31] Recent studies have shown a better prognosis. One study reported a median survival time of 14.0 months with procarbazine and prednisone treatment compared with 0.62 months for dogs not receiving treatment.[37] Another study showed a median survival time of 930 days with use of cyclosporine or in combination with corticosteroids or ketoconazole.[36] A study comparing the use of lomustine and prednisolone with prednisolone alone yielded a median survival time of 457 days compared with 329 days, respectively. The difference in survival time between groups was not statistically significant.[38] A study evaluating the use of cytosine arabinoside and prednisone in 10 dogs with inflammatory brain disease of unknown cause indicated a median survival time of 531 days. The study included dogs with suspected GME as well as NME or NLE.[39]

NECROTIZING ENCEPHALITIS

NME is an inflammatory disease causing necrotic cystic lesions within the gray and white matter of the cerebrum. In pugs, Chihuahuas, Maltese terriers, shih tzu and papillon the necrotic condition is often adjacent to the cerebral gray-white matter junction. In the Yorkshire terrier, NLE causes necrotic white matter lesions in the cerebrum and typically inflammatory lesions in the brainstem and cerebellum. Because of the breed-specific variance in lesion location it is uncertain whether these diseases are variants of the same disease or different diseases.[40] NME and NLE have also been reported in the Pekingese and French bulldog.[40,41] Male and female, young to middle-aged dogs are typically affected; however, dogs as old as 10 years of age have been reported. Seizures are common. Mentation changes, circling, and placing deficits may also be seen. Vestibular signs may predominate when the brainstem is affected in NLE. CSF typically indicates a mononuclear pleocytosis with increased protein. However, at times CSF is normal. MRI helps confirm the location and presence of cavitative lesions. MRI may also differentiate the disease from GME. Lesions with NME are multifocal, asymmetric, and present at the gray-white matter junction. They are typically hyperintense on T2 and FLAIR imaging and isointense or hypointense on T1 imaging. Contrast enhancement is variable (**Fig. 9**). NLE lesions are typically asymmetric, multifocal, and affect the subcortical white matter. The lesions are hyperintense on T2 and FLAIR imaging and isointense or hypointense on T1 imaging. Contrast enhancement is also variable (**Fig. 10**).[32] Recommended treatment is prednisone at 1 mg/kg by mouth twice a day with a gradual reduction in dose if response to therapy occurs. The

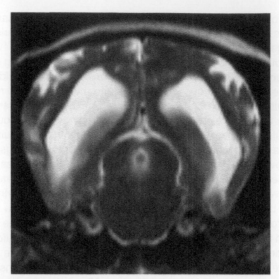

Fig. 9. Transverse T2-weighted MRI of a Chihuahua. Note the multifocal strongly hyperintense lesions affecting the cerebral gray matter consistent with NME. CSF indicated a WBC of 1/μL and a protein of 45 mg/dL.

prognosis for necrotizing encephalitis is poor. Mean survival time with corticosteroid treatment was 97 days in one study.[42] Dogs with necrotizing encephalitis may be less responsive to therapy than those treated for suspected GME.

INFECTIOUS DISEASES

Infectious diseases of the nervous system are more likely in puppies and kittens compared with adults. Poor suckling leading to malnutrition and incomplete transfer of maternal antibodies, difficult parturition, environmental stresses, and concurrent disease processes such as parvovirus can weaken the immune system, increasing

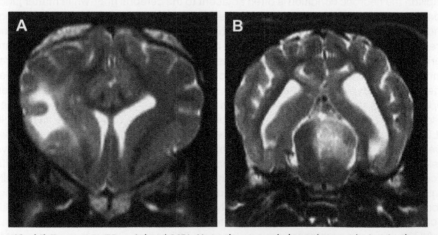

Fig. 10. (A) Transverse T2-weighted MRI. Note the strongly hyperintense lesion in the cerebral white matter. (B) Transverse T2-weighted MRI. A second hyperintense lesion is present in the midbrain. MRI is consistent with NLE.

the chance of bacterial meningoencephalitis. Animals with bacterial meningoencephalitis may have a fever or leukocytosis. Lethargy and apparent back pain may also be present. Thorough examination, abdominal ultrasound, and thoracic radiographs can identify a nidus of infection. The infection can arise from a dermal lesion or a recent surgical procedure with hematogenous spread to the CNS. Otitis media interna can spread centrally into the brain leading to bacterial meningitis.

CSF results with bacterial meningoencephalitis are neutrophilic. However, severe neutrophilic pleocytosis can also be seen with noninfectious inflammatory diseases such as steroid-responsive meningitis arteritis. MRI may identify meningeal enhancement, abscess formation, or otitis media interna consistent with an infectious process, making steroid-responsive meningitis arteritis less likely (**Figs. 11** and **12**). Culturing the CSF and/or urine may help identify a bacterial cause. Visualization of bacteria in the CSF allows a more definitive diagnosis of bacterial meningoencephalitis. *Staphylococcus*, *Escherichia coli*, *Streptococcus*, and various anaerobes are typically present in bacterial meningoencephalitis.[43] CNS penetration is often a consideration when choosing an antibiotic. At first, the compromised blood-brain barrier allows better penetration into the CNS. Once the blood barrier is intact, antibiotic penetration may be more difficult. Thus, a longer course of antibiotic therapy, higher dosages, or choosing an antibiotic that more reliably penetrates the CNS may be required. Chloramphenicol reaches high CNS concentrations, but is not typically used because of the potential adverse effects, particularly in neonates. Doxycycline penetrates the CNS, but its bacteriostatic nature and concerns for its use in young animals should be considered. Trimethoprim/sulfa also reaches high CNS concentrations, but concerns regarding potential adverse effects have also limited its use. Amoxicillin/clavulanic acid is broad spectrum, but reaches low CSF concentrations when the blood-brain barrier is intact. Fluoroquinolones are good choices for *Staphylococcus* and *E coli*, but have variable effects on *Streptococcus* and also reach low CSF concentrations.[44]

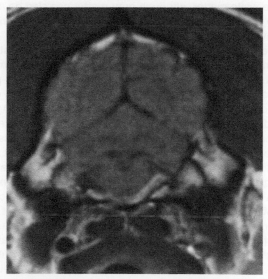

Fig. 11. Transverse T1-weighted postcontrast MRI. Contrast enhancement is present in the ventrolateral brainstem consistent with an infectious process rather than steroid-responsive meningitis arteritis.

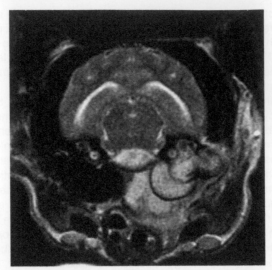

Fig. 12. Transverse T2-weighted MRI. Hyperintense material is present in the tympanic cavity, in the soft tissue surrounding the tympanic bulla, and in the ventral brainstem. Otitis media interna has spread centrally into the brainstem.

DISTEMPER

Canine distemper virus (CDV), a single-stranded RNA Morbillivirus, is typically spread through an aerosol route. CDV is epitheliotropic. The respiratory system is initially infected, with subsequent spread to the CNS, integument, bladder, and intestinal tract. CDV enters the nervous system through CSF or crosses the blood-brain barrier via infected mononuclear cells. Multifocal lesions are common. Primary demyelination often occurs in the white matter, although gray matter can also be affected. Areas of the brain that are commonly affected include the cerebellum, periventricular white matter, optic pathways, and spinal cord.[45]

Clinical signs are typically seen in dogs less than 1 year old. Persistent viral infection can lead to a chronic form, so-called old-dog distemper. Outbreaks may occur, particularly in animal shelters, caused by crowded conditions, diverse populations, and stress. A study in a Florida animal shelter indicated that only 43.2% of dogs admitted into the shelter had a protective antibody titer (PAT) for distemper. Age and whether a dog was neutered were associated with a PAT. Seventy-five percent of dogs more than 2 years old had a PAT compared with only 17.1% of dogs less than 1 year old. Neutered dogs were 8.3 times more likely to have a PAT than intact dogs.[46] Vaccination has reduced the incidence, but 30% of cases occur in vaccinated dogs.[47] Neurologic signs are typically focal despite multifocal lesions. Seizures and myoclonus are the most common neurologic signs. Brainstem, cerebellar, and myelopathic signs may also be seen.[48] Myoclonus may be caused by hyperexcitability of the lower motor neuron. It may persist during sleep, but disappears with anesthesia.[49]

The diagnosis of CDV is often based on clinical signs. The combination of neurologic abnormalities, particularly myoclonus, with extraneural signs should lead to a high suspicion of CDV. Extraneural signs are common and include pneumonia, enteritis, conjunctivitis, rhinitis, discolored teeth, and hyperkeratosis of the nasal planum and foot pads.[47] Pulmonary infiltrates are often identified by thoracic radiographs.[48] CSF often identifies a mononuclear pleocytosis, but albuminocytologic disassociation or normal CSF analysis can occur.[47] Serology is not typically helpful because of prior vaccination or previous subclinical infection. Severe CDV infection can sometimes have a low titer from immunosuppression. Direct immunofluorescence testing of conjunctival, vaginal, and nasal smears can confirm CDV only within 3 weeks of infection.[50] Polymerase chain reaction (PCR) testing can be helpful. PCR testing may be done on CSF, blood, conjunctiva, or urine. Reverse transcriptase PCR (RTPCR) is considered to be the best antemortem method used to detect CDV. RTPCR detected CDV RNA in 88% of infected dogs via whole blood or CSF testing and in 86% of infected dogs via serum testing. In one study, 22 of 22 dogs tested positive when PCR testing was done on the urine. Twelve asymptomatic dogs tested negative. Vaccine virus can be identified for a couple of days after vaccination.[51]

The prognosis for distemper infections is variable. Severely affected dogs are likely to die, whereas mildly affected dogs may recover. Supportive care is the mainstay of therapy. Anticonvulsants should be used to treat seizures, antibiotics for pneumonia, and intravenous fluids to maintain hydration. Concurrent toxoplasma infection may occur and, if present, should be treated.[52]

NEOSPOROSIS

Neospora caninum, a protozoal parasite, is a primary CNS and neuromuscular pathogen in dogs. Pneumonia, encephalitis, myocarditis, hepatitis, and myonecrosis are the predominant lesions in neonates. Ninety-two percent of affected dogs are less than 1 year old. Transplacental transmission is the major route of infection. An ascending paralysis is typically the presenting sign with possible progression to the cervical, brainstem, and cerebellar regions. Polyradiculoneuritis and polymyositis may result in hyperextension of the pelvic limbs. Creatine kinase can be increased when a polymyositis is present. CSF abnormalities typically include a mononuclear pleocytosis. The diagnosis can be supported via serum immunofluorescence antibody (IFA) titers. Affected dogs have IFA titers greater than 1:200. However, clinically normal dogs can have titers as high 1:800. Tachyzoites can be identified in cells from CSF, dermal lesions, and bronchial lavage.[53] PCR of the CSF was positive in 4 of 5 dogs in one report.[54] Clindamycin 10 to 15 mg/kg by mouth every 12 hours for 4 weeks is typically used for neosporosis therapy,[52] although trimethoprim sulfonamide 15 to 20 mg/kg by mouth every 12 hours may also be used alone or concurrently with clindamycin. Clindamycin is effective against tachyzoites, but is likely ineffective against encysted bradyzoites. Despite clinical improvement the *N caninum* infection is not cleared from the body.[55] The prognosis is considered poor,[53] but successful treatment is possible. Delayed therapy, muscle fibrosis, and pelvic limb hyperextension are considered poor prognostic indicators.[54]

TOXOPLASMOSIS

Toxoplasma gondii is a protozoal parasite that is transmitted via ingestion of sporulated oocysts transplacentally or in undercooked meats.[56] Cats are the definitive host. The most severe signs are caused by transplacental infection in kittens. Kittens may be stillborn or die within weeks. Pulmonary, CNS, cardiac, pancreatic, hepatic, and ocular lesions are common in clinically infected cats. Brain lesions are common, although neurologic signs are absent in many affected cats.[57] Muscle involvement is uncommon in cats.[58] Toxoplasma encephalitis occurs in up to 30% of people with acquired immune deficiency syndrome.[56] Histopathologic brain lesions are common, with 53 of 55 histologically examined cats having lesions in one study. The most common lesions were disseminated glial histiocytic granulomas and mononuclear perivascular cuffing. Despite the frequency of histologic lesions, neurologic signs in the study were uncommon. Only 7 of 100 infected cats had clinical neurologic abnormalities. Eighty percent of brains examined brains had *Toxoplasma* organisms identified.[57] Most clinical cases result from reactivated infections in cats older than 3 months of age.[58]

Positive serology can support the diagnosis. However 30% of cats and dogs have *T gondii* antibodies.[55,56] Positive immunoglobulin (Ig) M antibodies indicate recent infection and last for up to 12 weeks after inoculation. IgM antibodies typically are not seen in healthy cats and correlate more closely with disease. IgG antibodies support a more chronic infection.[56] CSF analysis in CNS toxoplasmosis typically shows a mixed pleocytosis and increased protein.[55] PCR testing can be done directly on CSF when toxoplasma is suspected. Clindamycin 10 to 12.5 mg/kg by mouth every 12 hours for 4 weeks is the treatment of choice.[55]

CRYPTOCOCCOSIS

Cryptococcus neoformans and *Cryptococcus gatti* are saprophytic yeastlike fungi. The characteristic heteropolysaccharide capsule provides virulence and resistance to desiccation.[59] Eight molecular types have been described. VN I, a type of *C neoformans,* is the most common type in dogs. VG III, a type of *C gatti*, is most common in cats.[60] Inhalation is the most likely route of infection. A predilection for the CNS occurs in both dogs and cats. Up to 55% of cats with cryptococcosis have CNS involvement.[61] No age predilection is present in cats, whereas affected dogs are typically less than 4 years of age.[62] CNS signs depend on lesion location. Cerebral involvement, particularly the olfactory bulb, is common, with seizures and obtundation being common signs. Vestibular involvement is common.[59] Systemic abnormalities are also common, including chorioretinitis; nasal discharge; skin lesions; hilar lymphadenopathy; and renal, hepatic, and splenic involvement.[59,63] Therefore a thorough fundic examination, thoracic radiographs, and abdominal ultrasound are recommended when cryptococcosis is suspected.

Serum latex agglutination (LA) testing is highly sensitive and specific. LA testing is 91.6% to 98% sensitive[64] and was 98% specific in one study.[61] Neurologic signs and a positive serum LA test suggest CNS cryptococcosis. Identification of organisms in the CSF or positive CSF LA testing confirms the diagnosis. Negative serum LA testing with positive yeast identification or positive LA results in the CSF is possible.[65] MRI results are variable. MRI may identify a gelatinous pseudocyst that is hypointense on T1 imaging and hyperintense on T2 imaging. The pseudocyst may have peripheral contrast enhancement. Meningeal, ependymal, or choroid plexus contrast enhancement may occur in other cases. An increased cellular/granulomatous response in dogs compared with cats may correlate with contrast enhancement patterns identified on MRI **(Fig. 13)**.[59,66]

Azole therapy is most commonly used for the treatment of cryptococcosis. Cryptococcosis is often treated successfully. Twenty-eight of 29 cats treated with fluconazole had successful outcomes.[67] However, CNS involvement likely decreases the prognosis. Fluconazole has good CSF penetration and thus is recommended in CNS cryptococcosis. Fluconazole 25 to 50 mg by mouth twice a day is typically used in the cat and 2.5 to 10 mg/kg per day divided twice a day is used in the dog.[59]

Itraconazole 5 to 10 mg/kg per day may also be used. Successful outcomes occurred in 56% of cats and improvement was seen in 29% of cats treated with itraconazole in one study.[68] Itraconazole is highly protein bound, insoluble in fluids, and is larger than fluconazole. It does not seem to cross the blood CSF barrier in detectable

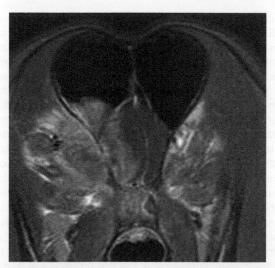

Fig. 13. MRI of a 1.5-year-old German shepherd dog with CNS cryptococcosis in the olfactory bulb and nasal cavity. Transverse postcontrast T1-weighted image. Marked contrast enhancement is present with a midline shift of the falx cerebri.

amounts.[69] Itraconazole may successfully treat CNS cryptococcosis by crossing an inflamed blood-brain barrier or via drug accumulation within the highly lipid brain.[70] In immunosuppressed people, initial treatment of cryptococcal meningitis has been a combination of intravenous amphotericin B and oral flucytosine. After 2 weeks of therapy, people are switched to azole therapy. *Cryptococcus* is susceptible to amphotericin B. However, the duration of use is limited because of poor CNS penetration and the potential for renal toxicity.[71] Daily monitoring of renal values is recommended when administering amphotericin B. Lipid-complexed amphotericin B has increased efficacy and is less nephrotoxic than standard amphotericin B.[59,70] Flucytosine 50 mg/kg by mouth every 8 hours in cats[44] penetrates well into the CSF, but should not be used as a single agent because resistance develops quickly.[72] Flucytosine can cause dermal eruptions in dogs.[62]

The prognosis for dogs and cats with cryptococcosis is considered worse when the CNS is involved. Remission of greater than 1 year occurred in only 32% of cats and dogs in one study. Abnormal mentation was associated with a poor outcome. Single-drug therapy versus Multiple-drug therapy did not significantly affect the outcome. The use of glucocorticoids improved survival time within the first 10 days.[66] CNS mycoses often cause inflammation and edema. Dying organisms can cause further inflammation and neurologic deterioration.[73] Glucocorticoids decrease inflammation and edema within the CNS. Thus, when MRI indicates significant brain edema or when significant neurologic deterioration occurs, the use of glucocorticoids is indicated. Dexamethasone sodium phosphate 0.1 mg/kg IV or subcutaneously every 12 hours followed by prednisone 0.5 mg/kg by mouth twice a day is used. Prednisone should be tapered over 1 to 2 weeks if possible because high doses or long-term use of corticosteroids to avoid immunosuppression.[59]

FIP

FIP is a common and fatal infectious feline disease caused by a mutant form of feline enteric corona virus.[74] A pyogranulomatous meningoencephalitis and meningomyelitis is seen with CNS involvement. The median age of cats with FIP affecting the CNS is 1 year.[75] The diagnosis of FIP can often be challenging. Cats with neurologic FIP may have weight loss, mentation changes, seizures, ataxia, and hyperesthesia. Anterior uveitis, hyphema and retinal hemorrhage may be identified on ophthalmologic examination.[74] Serum globulins are often increased.[76] Seronegative FIP may be seen in cats with low titers, acute fulminant disease less than 10 days, and from immune complex consumption.[77] MRI may identify periventricular changes consistent with ependymitis. The third and fourth ventricles are commonly affected. Secondary hydrocephalus may also be identified. CSF analysis indicates an increased protein value (mean 97.3 g/dL)[74] and a neutrophilic pleocytosis (mean 28 cells/μL).[75] CSF antibodies are likely of serum origin, but conflicting studies make the definitive antibody origin unknown.[74,75] A ratio of CSF antibodies/serum antibodies compared with CSF protein/serum total protein greater than 1 has typically suggested intrathecal antibody production.[74,75] However, a value greater than 1 does not necessarily imply active CNS infection.[75] Prednisolone therapy is typically given at immunosuppressive dosages (1–2 mg/kg by mouth every 12 hours or typically 5 mg per cat by mouth every 12 hours) to cats with neurologic FIP to decrease CNS inflammation and for immunosuppression, but the prognosis is ultimately poor.

EPILEPSY

Benign familial juvenile epilepsy has been reported in Lagotto Romagnolo dogs and is thought to be recessively inherited. Seizures are noted between 5 and 9 weeks of age. Seizures typically respond to anticonvulsant therapy. Discontinuation of anticonvulsants is often possible after several months of therapy. Seizure recurrence may occur in adulthood.[78]

Idiopathic epilepsy is classified as recurrent seizures without an apparent cause. Interictal neurologic examination is normal. Results of blood work, MRI, and CSF are all normal. Seizures typically are first noted between the ages of 1 and 5 years. Generalized tonic-clonic seizures are typically seen, although focal seizures are also possible. Idiopathic epilepsy is sometimes used to imply familial epilepsy because it is inherited in beagles, golden retrievers, Irish wolfhounds, English springer spaniels, Labrador retrievers, vizslas, Bernese mountain dogs, boxers, Belgian Tervurens, British Alsatians, Keeshonds, and standard poodles. Autosomal recessive inheritance is most common.[79] Anticonvulsant therapy is typically started when seizure frequency increases, particularly when 2 or more seizures occur within 6 months. A baseline period is helpful to determine the natural seizure frequency and can help assess response to anticonvulsant therapy. However, this baseline period should not be too long because early antiepileptic treatment may lead to better seizure control.[80] Patients with cluster seizures, status epilepticus, or secondary epilepsy should have anticonvulsant therapy started without delay. Anticonvulsant therapy is targeted to decrease the frequency and severity of seizures, increasing quality of life with as few adverse effects as possible.

ANTICONVULSANT CHOICES

The choice of anticonvulsant for maintenance therapy is tailored to each individual patient. The patient's age, medical history, potential for adverse effects, severity of the seizure disorder, and client concerns must all be considered. In patients with a history of cluster seizures, status epilepticus, or a progressive cause for seizures, the author typically chooses phenobarbital given its increased efficacy compared with other anticonvulsant options. Otherwise, in young patients with a less severe seizure disorder, the author often chooses either potassium bromide or levetiracetam given the decreased chance of hepatotoxicity. If a client is unable to consistently give medication multiple times a day, then starting with potassium bromide is reasonable. However, for dogs with a history of gastrointestinal issues, the author typically avoids potassium bromide. Although each medication has its benefits and risks, there is not a universal perfect anticonvulsant. Each medication may need to be adjusted for optimal seizure control or because of potential adverse effects. Monotherapy is typically preferred for initial therapy. However, when the seizure disorder is refractory to monotherapy, then multidrug therapy is indicated in the pursuit of adequate seizure control. It is important to educate clients about the goals of anticonvulsant therapy (improved seizure control with minimal to no adverse effects), potential adverse effects, and potential future need for multidrug therapy.

PHENOBARBITAL

Phenobarbital historically has been the first-line treatment of seizures in dogs and cats. Phenobarbital is the most efficacious anticonvulsant, with one study reporting efficacy in 90% of suspected epileptic dogs.[81] Phenobarbital increases the seizure threshold and decreases the spread to surrounding neurons. It enhances the inhibitory postsynaptic effects of gamma-aminobutyric acid (GABA), inhibits glutamate activity, and decreases calcium flux across neuronal membranes. Peak levels are achieved 4 to 6 hours after oral administration and its half-life ($T_{1/2}$) is 1.5 to 3 days. Phenobarbital metabolism increases with chronic therapy.[82] Phenobarbital is typically started at 2.5 to 3 mg/kg by mouth every 12 hours. The dose is then adjusted based on clinical response, adverse effects, and serum levels. Adverse effects include sedation, ataxia, polyphagia, polyuria/polydypsia (PU/PD), and increased liver enzymes. The potential for liver failure increases at serum levels of 35 to 40 µg/mL (therapeutic range, 15–40 µg/mL). Routine liver monitoring is recommended.[82] Increases in alkaline phosphatase (ALP), alanine aminotransferase (ALT) and gamma glutamyl transferase (GGT) can result from enzyme induction rather than hepatic injury. Bile acid testing, bilirubin, and abdominal ultrasound were not affected by phenobarbital therapy in one study. Thus, bile acid testing, bilirubin, and abdominal ultrasound can help assess liver disease in dogs receiving phenobarbital.[83] Larger increases in ALT compared with ALP are concerning because it also suggests hepatic disease. Hepatotoxicity can improve as the phenobarbital dose is lowered or withdrawn. However, with advanced liver disease, the effects can be irreversible and potentially fatal.[80] Evaluating CBC and chemistry 2 to 4 weeks after starting therapy, 3 months later, and then every 6 months can be helpful. Bile acid testing should also be considered periodically or if hepatic enzymes are increasing. Phenobarbital's shorter $T_{1/2}$, compared with bromide, allows quicker manipulation of plasma levels, making it a good choice for dogs with frequent seizures.

Phenobarbital has been associated with rare congenital defects and bleeding problems in neonates. Although caution is recommended, phenobarbital is considered likely to be safer than other anticonvulsants. Small amounts are excreted into maternal milk and thus may affect nursing animals.[44]

Assessment of hypothyroidism is difficult in dogs receiving phenobarbital. Total T4 (TT4) and freeT4 (FT4) values may be significantly decreased in dogs receiving phenobarbital. Total T3 changes minimally and thyroid-stimulating hormone (TSH) increases after several months of phenobarbital therapy. Serum cholesterol also increases after phenobarbital administration. It is unclear whether the decrease in TT4 and FT4 is clinically significant. Increased thyroxine monoiodination to T3 at the cellular level may occur, compensating for hypothyroxinemia. If so, TT4, FT4, and

TSH values are meaningless.[84] TT4 values return to normal within 6 weeks of pheno-barbital withdrawal. FT4 values may remain decreased for 10 weeks after cessation of phenobarbital therapy.[85]

BROMIDE

Bromide has also been a popular first-choice or second-choice anticonvulsant. Bromide was effective in 72% of epileptic dogs in one study[86] and 74% in another study.[81] Bromide hyperpolarizes the neuron through its replacement of chloride ions.[82] Bromide has a $T_{1/2}$ of 21 to 24 days and is excreted by the kidneys.[80] Increased dietary salt intake increases renal excretion. Adverse effects of bromide include seda-tion, ataxia, PU/PD, polyphagia, gastrointestinal effects,[82] and a possible association with pancreatitis.[80] The lack of hepatic metabolism makes potassium bromide, 40 mg/kg/d in food, a good choice for young dogs. The therapeutic range is 1.0 to 3.0 mg/mL. If dogs are in status epilepticus or have cluster seizures, the long $T_{1/2}$ of bromide can make it more difficult to use effectively. In these situations, a drug with a shorter $T_{1/2}$ may be a better choice. A loading dose of potassium bromide can be given at 450 to 600 mg/kg by mouth total over the course of 5 days.[82] Adverse effects are more com-mon when using a loading dose. Bromide should not be given to cats because it causes pneumonitis in cats. The pneumonitis is typically reversible once bromide ther-apy is stopped.[80] The reproductive safety of bromide has not been determined.[44]

LEVETIRACETAM

Levetiracetam has become increasing popular in the past decade. A few studies with limited power have indicated 56% to 64% response to adjunctive levetiracetam ther-apy for epilepsy[87,88] as well as for emergency treatment of status epilepticus and clus-ter seizures.[89] Levetiracetam binds synaptic vesicular protein SV2A. Levetiracetam may prevent hypersynchronization of burst firing and seizure propagation. The $T_{1/2}$ is 4 hours in dogs and 5 hours in cats. Initial dosing was recommended at 10 to 20 mg/kg by mouth 3 times a day. However, a honeymoon effect was noted. After several months of therapy, seizure control was lost.[87] This honeymoon phenomenon and pharmacokinetic evaluation has led to a recommended starting dose of 20 mg/kg by mouth 3 times a day.[90] An extended-release formulation is now also available and is dosed at 20 mg/kg by mouth twice a day. The extended-release tablets are not suit-able for small dogs or cats because the tablets should not be cut. The adverse effects of levetiracetam seem minimal with sedation/ataxia occurring uncommonly. Sixty-six percent of the drug is excreted unchanged through the kidneys. The cytochrome P 450 system does not seem to be involved. However, concurrent phenobarbital admin-istration has been shown to decrease levetiracetam $T_{1/2}$ and decreases levetiracetam blood levels. Thus dogs on both phenobarbital and levetiracetam concurrently may require higher dosages of levetiracetam.[91] Levetiracetam is excreted into maternal milk and so should be used with caution in nursing animals. Levetiracetam should be used with caution in pregnant animals because high dosages have increased embryofetal mortality in rabbits and rats.[44]

ZONISAMIDE

Zonisamide is a sulfonamide-based anticonvulsant drug that has also become popular in the past decade. As with levetiracetam, a few reports with limited patient numbers have been published. One study indicated that 9 of 11 refractory epileptic dogs responded to zonisamide therapy in the first 8 months of therapy. However, only 6 of 11 responded after 17 months of therapy.[92] Another study indicated that 7 of 12 refractory epileptic dogs responded to zonisamide therapy.[93] Zonisamide monotherapy was effective in 6 of 10 epileptic dogs in another report.[94] Zonisamide blocks voltage-dependent sodium channels and T-type calcium channels. Its $T_{1/2}$ is about 15 hours in the dog and 35 hours in cats. Zonisamide is metabolized by hepatic microsomal enzymes and is also renally excreted. Its $T_{1/2}$ is reduced with concurrent phenobarbital administration. Zonisamide is administered 5 to 10 mg/kg by mouth twice a day in dogs, with the higher dose range for dogs also receiving phenobarbital. Cats are given 5 to 10 mg/kg by mouth every 24 hours, because of the longer $T_{1/2}$. Zonisamide is typically well tolerated, with anorexia, sedation, and ataxia being the most common adverse effects.[80] Acute hepatopathy within 3 weeks of starting zonisamide therapy has recently been reported in 2 dogs.[95,96] Renal tubular acidosis has also been reported recently. Acid-base changes resolved after discontinuation of zonisamide.[97] When zonisamide was given to pregnant dogs, ventricular septal defects, cardiomegaly, and valvular and arterial anomalies occurred. Thus zonisamide is not recommended for use in pregnant animals. It is unknown whether zonisamide is excreted into maternal milk.[44]

GABAPENTIN

Gabapentin binds voltage-gated calcium channels and decreases intracellular calcium influx. It is excreted unchanged by the kidneys with about 30% to 40% hepatic metabolism in dogs.[98] Gabapentin's maximum absorption occurs within 2 hours of administration. The $T_{1/2}$ is 3 to 4 hours in dogs[99] and 3 hours in cats.[100] The initial dose is 10 mg/kg by mouth 3 times a day. Six of 11 refractory epileptic dogs responded to gabapentin therapy in one study.[99] Sedation and ataxia are the most common adverse effects.[80] The liquid formulation contains xylitol and thus should not be given to dogs. Dogs requiring liquid or small doses should have the drug compounded so that it does not contain xylitol. Gabapentin has been teratogenic in mice, rats, and rabbits and should thus be used with caution or avoided in pregnant animals. Gabapentin is excreted through maternal milk. However, the amount that is excreted is not thought to be clinically significant.[44]

PREGABALIN

Pregabalin is a GABA analogue structurally similar to gabapentin. Pregabalin has a higher affinity for the alpha-2-delta subunit of neuronal voltage-gated calcium channels than does gabapentin. The $T_{1/2}$ of pregabalin is 7 hours in dogs[98] and 10.4 hours in cats.[101] Pregabalin is administered at 2 to 4 mg/kg by mouth 2 to 3 times a day. Seven of 11 refractory epileptic dogs responded to pregabalin therapy in one study. Adverse effects included sedation and ataxia and were common. Thus, a starting dose of 2 mg/kg by mouth 2 to 3 times a day with a gradual increase in dose by 1 mg/kg is recommended in dogs.[98] A dose of 1 to 2 mg/kg by mouth twice a day is recommended in cats.[101] Very high dosages of pregabalin given to pregnant rats and rabbits caused skeletal malformations in offspring. Pregabalin is also excreted into maternal milk.[44]

FELBAMATE

Felbamate enhances the inhibitory effects of GABA, blocks voltage-dependent sodium channels, and blocks N-methyl-D-aspartate receptors.[80,102] The $T_{1/2}$ in dogs is 5 to 6 hours and is administered at a starting dose of 15 mg/kg[80] to 20 mg/kg[102] by mouth 3 times a day. Doses as high as 70 mg/kg by mouth 3 times a day may be required in some dogs. Felbamate can cause aplastic anemia and fatal hepatopathy in people, thus its use is limited. In dogs, about 30% of felbamate undergoes hepatic metabolism with the rest excreted unchanged in the urine. Adverse effects in dogs include hepatic effects, mild thrombocytopenia, and leukopenia.[80,102] Blood dyscrasias were reversible with stopping felbamate therapy.[102] Felbamate is excreted into maternal milk. Although no overt teratogenic effects have been documented, caution is recommended in pregnant animals.[44]

BENZODIAZEPINES

Benzodiazepines are potent anticonvulsants that enhance the inhibitory effects of GABA. The $T_{1/2}$ of diazepam is 3.2 hours in dogs and about 15 to 20 hours in cats. The longer $T_{1/2}$ of diazepam in cats makes it a possible candidate for long-term anticonvulsant therapy. However, the use of oral diazepam is limited because of the potential risk of severe/fatal liver disease in cats. Strict monitoring is required if diazepam is used orally in cats. Tolerance develops with maintenance use of benzodiazepines. Thus the short duration of action in dogs and the development of tolerance limit the use of benzodiazepines to the emergency setting.[80,82] Diazepam at 0.5 mg/kg IV or 1 to 2 mg/kg rectally is recommended for immediate treatment of seizures. The absorption of benzodiazepines when administered rectally is variable, resulting in questionable efficacy. Concurrent phenobarbital administration increases the metabolism of diazepam. Thus, the higher dose range is recommended for rectal diazepam when dogs are concurrently receiving phenobarbital therapy. Diazepam 0.5 mg/kg/h may be administered as a constant-rate infusion (CRI). The dose is then titrated based on seizure control and sedation.[80] Midazolam is water soluble and is a good choice for emergency treatment when a CRI is needed through a peripheral catheter or via intramuscular injection. Midazolam's $T_{1/2}$ in dogs is 77 minutes.[103] A dose of 0.07 to 0.2 mg/kg is recommended as an intravenous or intramuscular bolus for immediate seizure control and a dosage of 0.05 to 0.5 mg/kg/h when given as a CRI. When a benzodiazepine has been used to stop the acute seizure, it is important to also administer a longer acting anticonvulsant to prevent further seizures.[80]

Diazepam causes congenital abnormalities when given in the first trimester of pregnancy and should be avoided if possible in pregnant animals. Benzodiazepines and metabolites are excreted into maternal milk and can thus affect nursing animals.[44]

Clorazepate is metabolized to nordiazepam and has a $T_{1/2}$ of 4 to 6 hours in dogs. Tolerance does not develop as readily compared with diazepam. Clorazepate may be helpful in short-term control of breakthrough seizures.[82] A dose of 0.5 to 1 mg/kg by mouth 2 to 3 times a day is recommended.[44,82] Clorazepate increases phenobarbital levels. Serum phenobarbital levels should be monitored with its use 2 and 4 weeks after starting clorazepate therapy.[82] Clorazepate should be used with extreme caution in aggressive animals. The metabolite nordiazepam is distributed into milk and thus may affecting nursing animals.[44]

The use of acepromazine in dogs with a history of seizures has commonly not been recommended because of a possible decrease in the seizure threshold with its use. However, evidence to warrant a contraindication for the use of acepromazine in patients with seizures is lacking. The use of acepromazine in patients with seizures is unlikely to result in seizures. A retrospective study evaluated 36 dogs with a history of seizures that were given acepromazine for sedation or as a preanesthetic. None of the 36 dogs had seizures within 16 hours of use.[104]

THERAPEUTIC MONITORING

Therapeutic levels and toxic levels are guidelines extrapolated from people. These ranges are based on population statistics and may not accurately reflect whether an individual canine or feline patient is controlled. Nonetheless, they can be helpful in optimizing anticonvulsant therapy, assessing risk factors of therapy, and helping to gauge when a second anticonvulsant may be needed. Determining anticonvulsant levels is most beneficial when (1) a dose change is needed because of inadequate seizure control or toxicity. The formula (desired blood level/current blood level) times the current dose equals the newly recommended dose (2) A refractory patient becomes controlled, which allows the identification of a therapeutic level for that patient, provided the seizure disorder does not worsen. (3) The patient is sensitive to the toxic effects of the anticonvulsant (most commonly bromide). Obtaining a blood level as soon as clinical signs of toxicity abate identifies the toxic level for that patient. Evaluation of blood levels may not be important when patients are currently and historically well controlled and free of adverse effects. Patients receiving phenobarbital should ideally have a level obtained once they reach steady state given the risk of hepatotoxicity at levels greater than 35 μg/mL. In addition, serial phenobarbital levels every 6 to 12 months can be of benefit if hepatic metabolism changes. Peak and trough phenobarbital levels were recommended in the past. However, only 9% of patients receiving phenobarbital had a clinically significant (>30%) change between peak and trough levels in one study. Thus a single sample is typically sufficient.[105] Identifying the timing of sample collection relative to dosing can be helpful when the level is in the high reference range so that toxicity can be avoided. Therapeutic levels for levetiracetam, zonisamide, and pregabalin are unknown for dogs at this time. Thus, routine monitoring of levels is typically not done with usage of these drugs. Bromide levels are affected by Cl^-. Increased dietary Cl^- or intravenous fluids containing Cl^- increase renal excretion of bromide and thus lower serum bromide levels. A patient receiving bromide therapy may lose seizure control as a result of a change in diet or intravenous fluids. In contrast, a decrease in dietary Cl^- may lead to toxicity (sedation and ataxia) as renal bromide excretion is reduced and serum bromide levels subsequently increase. Thus, dietary changes should be minimized in patients receiving bromide therapy.

When transitioning from one anticonvulsant to another, several factors may influence the recommendations for the transition. If significant adverse effects are not apparent, then it is reasonable to add the additional drug while continuing the initial anticonvulsant at the maintenance dose. If the initial anticonvulsant drug is to be withdrawn it should be tapered over the course of several months because it is often difficult to definitively know how effective the initial drug was. Weaning the initial drug over several months may help prevent withdrawal seizures. If sedation or ataxia is noted with the addition of the new anticonvulsant, either drug may be tapered to limit adverse effects. If seizure control is successful without adverse effects, maintenance therapy with multiple drugs may be warranted and thus the initial drug may not be withdrawn. If a second or third drug is implemented because of adverse effects, tapering the drug with the most likely adverse effects is recommended. If adverse effects are of mild to moderate concern then tapering a drug such as phenobarbital may be done every 2 to 4 weeks by 25% each time. Potassium bromide may be reduced more quickly at times because of its longer $T_{1/2}$. Rapid tapering or withdrawal is necessary when adjusting medications because of severe adverse effects from existing therapy. In this situation, the existing therapy should be stopped immediately or over the course of a few days. It is important to concurrently start another anticonvulsant with a shorter $T_{1/2}$ so that steady state is rapidly achieved. Furthermore, the additional drug should have a different profile of adverse effects.

REFERENCES

1. Mehl ML, Kyles AE, Hardie EM, et al. Evaluation of ameroid ring constrictors for treatment for single extrahepatic portsosystemic shunts in dogs: 168 cases (1196-1991). J Am Vet Med Assoc 2005;226:2020–30.
2. Tisdall PL, Hunt GB, Youmans KR, et al. Neurological dysfunction in dogs following attenuation of congenital extrahepatic portosystemic shunts. J Small Anim Pract 2000;41:539–46.
3. Podell M. Neurologic manifestations of systemic disease. In: Ettinger SJ, editor. Textbook of veterinary internal medicine. 6th edition. St Louis (MO): Elsevier; 2005. p. 798–802.
4. Ruland K, Fischer A, Hartmann K. Sensitivity and specificity of fasting ammonia and serum bile acids in the diagnosis of portosystemic shunts in dogs and cats. Vet Clin Pathol 2010;39:57–64.
5. D'Anjou MA, Pennick D, Cornejo L, et al. Ultrasonographic diagnosis of portosystemic shunting in dogs and cats. Vet Radiol Ultrasound 2004;45: 424–37.
6. Berent AC, Weisse C. Hepatic vascular anomalies. In: Ettinger SJ, editor. Textbook of veterinary internal medicine. 7th edition. St Louis (MO): Elsevier; 2010. p. 1649–72.
7. Greenhalgh SN, Dunning MD, McKinley TJ, et al. Comparison of survival after surgical or medical treatment in dogs with a congenital portosystemic shunt. J Am Vet Med Assoc 2010;236:1215–20.
8. Fryer KJ, Levine JM, Peycke LE, et al. Incidence of postoperative seizures with and without levetiracetam pretreatment in dogs undergoing portosystemic shunt attenuation. J Vet Intern Med 2011;25:1379–84.
9. Summers BA, Cummings JF, De Lahunta A. Malformations of the central nervous system. In: Veterinary neuropathology. St Louis (MO): Mosby; 1995. p. 68–94.
10. Wunschmann A, Oglesbee M. Periventricular changes associated with canine hydrocephalus. Vet Pathol 2001;38(1):67–73.
11. Zabka TS, Lavely JA, Higgins RJ. Primary intra-axial leiomyosarcoma with obstructive hydrocephalus in a young dog. J Comp Pathol 2004;131:334–7.
12. Hoskins JD. Clinical evaluation of the kitten: from birth to eight weeks of age. Compend Contin Educ Pract Vet 1990;12(9):1215–25.
13. Saito M, Olby NJ, Spaulding K, et al. Relationship among basilar artery resistance index, degree of ventriculomegaly, and clinical signs in hydrocephalic dogs. Vet Radiol Ultrasound 2003;44(6):687–94.
14. Harrington ML, Bagley RS, Moore MP. Hydrocephalus. Vet Clin North Am Small Anim Pract 1996;26(4):843–56.
15. Nykamp S, Scrivani P, De Lahunta A, et al. Chronic subdural hematomas and hydrocephalus in a dog. Vet Radiol Ultrasound 2001;42(6):511–4.
16. Lavely JA. Pediatric neurology of the dog and cat. Vet Clin North Am Small Anim Pract 2006;36:475–501.
17. Lindvall-Axelsson M, Hedner P, Owman C. Corticosteroid action on choroids plexus: reduction in Na-K ATPase activity, choline transport capacity, and rate of CSF formation. Exp Brain Res 1989;77:605–10.
18. Javaheri S, Corbett WS, Simbartl LA, et al. Different effects of omeprazole and Sch 28080 on canine cerebrospinal fluid production. Brain Res 1997;754:321–4.

19. Biel M, Kramer M, Forterre F, et al. Outcome of ventriculoperitoneal shunt implantation for treatment of congenital internal hydrocephalus in dogs and cats: 36 cases (2001–2009). J Am Vet Med Assoc 2013;242:948–58.
20. Shihab N, Davies E, Kenny PJ, et al. Treatment of hydrocephalus with ventriculoperitoneal shunting in twelve dogs. Vet Surg 2011;40:477–84.
21. de Stefani A, de Risio L, Platt SR, et al. Surgical technique, postoperative complications and outcome in 14 dogs treated for hydrocephalus by ventriculoperitoneal shunting. Vet Surg 2011;40:183–91.
22. Kestle J, Drake J, Milner R, et al. Long term follow-up data from the shunt design trial. Pediatr Neurosurg 2000;33:230–6.
23. Abramson CJ, Platt SR, Jakobs C, et al. L-2 hydroxyglutaric aciduria in Staffordshire bull terriers. J Vet Intern Med 2003;17:551–6.
24. Garosi LS, Penderis J, McConnell JF, et al. L-2 hydroxyglutaric aciduria in a West Highland white terrier. Vet Rec 2005;156:145–7.
25. Sanchez-Masian DF, Artuch R, Mascort J, et al. L-2-hydroxyglutaric aciduria in two female Yorkshire terriers. J Am Anim Hosp Assoc 2012;48(5):366–71.
26. Penderis J, Calvin J, Abramson C, et al. L-2-hydroxyglutaric aciduria: characterization of the molecular defect in a spontaneous canine model. J Med Genet 2007;44:334–40.
27. Platt S, McGrotty YL, Abramson CJ, et al. Refractory seizures associated with an organic aciduria in a dog. J Am Anim Hosp Assoc 2007;43:163–7.
28. Saito M, Sharp NJ, Kortz GD, et al. Magnetic resonance imaging features of lissencephaly in 2 Lhasa apsos. Vet Radiol Ultrasound 2002;43(4):331–7.
29. Zaki FA. Lissencephaly in Lhasa apso dogs. J Am Vet Med Assoc 1976;169: 1165–8.
30. Greene CE, Vandevelde M, Braund K. Lissencephaly in two Lhasa apso dogs. J Am Vet Med Assoc 1976;169(4):405–10.
31. Muñana KR, Luttgen PJ. Prognostic factors for dogs with granulomatous meningoencephalomyelitis: 42 cases (1982-1996). J Am Vet Med Assoc 1998;212(2): 1902–6.
32. Schatzberg SJ. Idiopathic granulomatous and necrotizing inflammatory disorders of the canine central nervous system. Vet Clin North Am Small Anim Pract 2010;40:101–20.
33. Lamb CR, Croson PJ, Cappello R, et al. Magnetic resonance imaging findings in 25 dogs with inflammatory cerebrospinal fluid. Vet Radiol Ultrasound 2005; 46(1):17–22.
34. Cherubini GB, Platt SR, Anderson TJ, et al. Characteristics of magnetic resonance images of granulomatous meningoencephalomyelitis in 11 dogs. Vet Rec 2006;159:110–5.
35. Cuddon PA, Coates JR, Murray M. New treatments for granulomatous meningoencephalomyelitis. In Proceedings 20th ACVIM. Dallas (TX): 2002. p. 319–21.
36. Adamo PF, Rylander H, Adams WM. Ciclosporin use in multi-drug therapy for meningoencephalomyelitis of unknown aetiology in dogs. J Small Anim Pract 2007;48(9):486–96.
37. Coates JR, Barone G, Dewey CW, et al. Procarbazine as adjunctive treatment of dogs with presumptive antemortem diagnosis of granulomatous meningoencephalomyelitis: 21 cases (1998-2004). J Vet Intern Med 2007;21:100–6.
38. Flegel T, Boettcher IC, Matiasek K, et al. Comparison of oral administration of lomustine and prednisolone or prednisolone alone as treatment for granulomatous meningoencephalomyelitis or necrotizing encephalitis in dogs. J Am Vet Med Assoc 2011;238:337–45.

39. Zarfoss M, Schatzberg S, Venator K, et al. Combined cytosine arabinoside and prednisone therapy for meningoencephalitis of unknown aetiology in 10 dogs. J Small Anim Pract 2006;47:588–95.

40. Higgins RJ, Dickinson PJ, Kube SA, et al. Necrotizing meningoencephalitis in 5 Chihuahua dogs. Vet Pathol 2008;45(3):336–46.

41. Park ES, Uchida K, Nakayama H. Comprehensive immunohistochemical studies on canine necrotizing meningoencephalitis (NME), necrotizing leukoencephalitis (NLE), and granulomatous meningoencephalomyelitis (GME). Vet Pathol 2012;49:682–92.

42. Levine JM, Fosgate GT, Porter B, et al. Epidemiology of necrotizing meningoencephalitis in pug dogs. J Vet Intern Med 2008;22:961–8.

43. Irwin PJ, Parry BW. Streptococcal meningoencephalitis in a dog. J Am Anim Hosp Assoc 1999;35:417–22.

44. Plumb DC. Veterinary drug handbook. 7th edition. Ames (IA): Wiley Blackwell; 2011.

45. Vandevelde M, Zurbriggen A. Demyelination in canine distemper virus infection: a review. Acta Neuropathol 2005;109:56–68.

46. Lechner ES, Crawford PC, Levy JK, et al. Prevalence of protective antibody titers for canine distemper virus and canine parvovirus in dogs entering a Florida animal shelter. J Am Vet Med Assoc 2010;236:1317–21.

47. Koutinas AF, Polizopoulou ZS, Baumgaertner W, et al. Relation of clinical signs to pathological changes in 19 cases of canine distemper encephalomyelitis. J Comp Pathol 2002;126:47–56.

48. Moritz A, Frisk AL, Baumgärtner W. The evaluation of diagnostic procedures for the detection of canine distemper virus infection. European Journal of Companion Animal Practice 2000;10:38–47.

49. Inada S. Electromyographic analysis of canine distemper myoclonus. Electromyogr Clin Neurophysiol 1989;29:323–31.

50. Jozwik A, Frymus T. Comparison of the immunofluorescence assay with RT-PCR and nested PCR in the diagnosis of canine distemper. Vet Res Commun 2005; 29:347–59.

51. Saito TB, Alfieri AA, Wosiacki SR, et al. Detection of canine distemper virus by reverse transcriptase-polymerase chain reaction in the urine of dogs with clinical signs of distemper encephalitis. Res Vet Sci 2006;80:116–9.

52. Dubey JP, Lappin MR. Toxoplasmosis and neosporosis. In: Greene CE, editor. Infectious diseases of the dog and cat. 2nd edition. Philadelphia: WB Saunders; 1998. p. 493–509.

53. Ruehlmann D, Podell M, Oglesbee M, et al. Canine neosporosis: a case report and literature review. J Am Anim Hosp Assoc 1995;31:174–83.

54. Garosi L, Dawson A, Couturier J, et al. Necrotizing cerebellitis and cerebellar atrophy caused by Neospora caninum infection: magnetic resonance imaging and clinicopathologic findings in seven dogs. J Vet Intern Med 2010;24:571–8.

55. Dubey JP, Lappin MR. Toxoplasmosis and neosporosis. In: Greene CE, editor. Infectious diseases of the dog and cat. 4th edition. St Louis (MO): Elsevier Saunders; 2012. p. 806–27.

56. Vollaire MR, Radecki SV, Lappin MR. Seroprevalence of Toxoplasma gondii antibodies in clinically ill cats in the United States. Am J Vet Res 2005;66(5):874–7.

57. Dubey JP, Carpenter JL. Histologically confirmed clinical toxoplasmosis in cats: 100 cases. J Am Vet Med Assoc 1993;203(1):1556–66.

58. Dickinson PJ, LeCouteur RA. Feline neuromuscular disorders. Vet Clin North Am Small Anim Pract 2004;34:1307–59.

59. Lavely J, Lipsitz D. Fungal infections of the central nervous system in the dog and cat. Clin Tech Small Anim Pract 2005;20:212–9.
60. Singer LM, Meyer W, Thompson GR, et al. Molecular epidemiology and antifungal susceptibility among *Cryptococcus* isolates from North American dogs and cats. J Vet Intern Med 2012;26(3):788–9.
61. Lester SJ, Kowalewich NJ, Bartlett KH, et al. Clinicopathologic features of an unusual outbreak of cryptococcosis in dogs, cats, ferrets, and a bird: 38 cases (January to July 2003). J Am Vet Med Assoc 2004;225:1716–22.
62. Kerl ME. Update on canine and feline fungal diseases. Vet Clin North Am Small Anim Pract 2003;33:721–47.
63. Berthelin CF, Legendre AM, Bailey CS, et al. Cryptococcosis of the nervous system in dogs, part 2: diagnosis, treatment, monitoring, and prognosis. Progr Vet Neurol 1994;5:136–46.
64. O'Toole TE, Sato AF, Rozanski EA. Cryptococcosis of the central nervous system in a dog. J Am Vet Med Assoc 2003;222:1722–6.
65. Stevenson TL, Dickinson PJ, Sturges BK, et al. Magnetic resonance imaging of intracranial cryptococcosis in dogs and cats. Proceedings ACVIM. Minneapolis (MN): 2004.
66. Sykes JE, Sturges BK, Cannon MS, et al. Clinical signs, imaging features, neuropathology, and outcome in cats and dogs with central nervous system cryptococcosis from California. J Vet Intern Med 2010;24:1427–38.
67. Malik R, Wigney DI, Muir DB, et al. Cryptococcosis in cats: clinical and mycological assessment of 29 cases and evaluation of treatment using orally administered fluconazole. J Med Vet Mycol 1992;30:133–44.
68. Medleau L, Jacobs GJ, Marks AM. Itraconazole for the treatment of *Cryptococcus* in cats. J Vet Intern Med 1995;9:39–42.
69. Perfect JR, Savani DV, Durack DT. Comparison of itraconazole and fluconazole in treatment of cryptococcal meningitis and *Candida* pyelonephritis in rabbits. Antimicrobial Agents Chemother 1986;29:579–83.
70. Grooters AM, Taboada J. Update on antifungal therapy. Vet Clin North Am Small Anim Pract 2003;33:749–58.
71. Davis LE. Fungal infections of the central nervous system infections. Neurol Clin 1999;17:761–81.
72. Slavoski LA, Tunkel AR. Therapy of fungal meningitis. Clin Neuropharmacol 1995;18:95–112.
73. Tiches D, Vite CH, Dayrell-Hart B, et al. A case of canine central nervous system cryptococcosis: management with fluconazole. J Am Anim Hosp Assoc 1998; 34:145–51.
74. Foley JE, Lapointe JM, Koblik P, et al. Diagnostic features of clinical neurologic feline infectious peritonitis. J Vet Intern Med 1998;12:415–23.
75. Boettcher IC, Steinberg T, Matiasek K, et al. Use of anti-coronavirus antibody testing of cerebrospinal fluid for diagnosis of feline infectious peritonitis involving the central nervous system in cats. J Am Vet Med Assoc 2007; 230(2):199–205.
76. Hartmann K, Binder C, Hirschberger J, et al. Comparison of different tests to diagnose feline infectious peritonitis. J vet Intern Med 2003;17:781–90.
77. Foley JE. Feline infectious peritonitis and feline enteric coronavirus. In: Ettinger S, Feldman E, editors. Textbook of veterinary internal medicine. 6th edition. St Louis (MO): Elsevier; 2005. p. 663–6.
78. Jokinen TS, Metsahonkala L, Bergamasco L, et al. Benign familial juvenile epilepsy in lagotto romagnolo dogs. J Vet Intern Med 2007;21:464–71.

79. Licht BG, Lin S, Luo Y, et al. Clinical characteristics and mode of inheritance of familial focal seizures in standard poodles. J Am Vet Med Assoc 2007;231(10): 1520–8.

80. Thomas WB. Idiopathic epilepsy in dogs and cats. Vet Clin North Am Small Anim Pract 2010;40:161–79.

81. Boothe DM, Dewey C, Carpenter DM. Comparison of phenobarbital with bromide as a first choice antiepileptic drug for treatment of epilepsy in dogs. J Am Vet Med Assoc 2012;240(9):1073–83.

82. Boothe DM. Anticonvulsant therapy in small animals. Vet Clin North Am Small Anim Pract 1998;28(2):411–48.

83. Müller PB, Taboada J, Hosgood G, et al. Effects of long-term phenobarbital treatment on the liver on dogs. J Vet Intern Med 2000;14:165–71.

84. Müller PB, Wolfsheimer KJ, Taboada J, et al. Effects of long term phenobarbital treatment on the thyroid and adrenal axis and adrenal function tests in dogs. J Vet Intern Med 2000;14:157–64.

85. Gieger TL, Hosgood G, Taboada J, et al. Thyroid function and serum hepatic enzyme activity in dogs after phenobarbital administration. J Vet Intern Med 2000;14(3):277–81.

86. Trepanier LA, Van Schoick A, Schwark WS, et al. Therapeutic serum drug concentrations in epileptic dogs treated with potassium bromide alone or in combination with other anticonvulsants: 122 cases (1992-1996). J Am Vet Med Assoc 1998;213(10):1449–53.

87. Volk HA, Matiasek LA, Feliu-Pascual AL, et al. The efficacy and tolerability of levetiracetam in pharmacoresistant epileptic dogs. Vet J 2008;176:310–9.

88. Muñana KR, Thomas WB, Inzana KD, et al. Evaluation of levetiracetam as adjunctive treatment for refractory canine epilepsy: a randomized, placebo-controlled, crossover trial. J Vet Intern Med 2012;26:341–8.

89. Hardy BT, Patterson EE, Cloyd JM, et al. Double-masked, placebo-controlled study of intravenous levetiracetam for the treatment of status epilepticus and acute repetitive seizures in dogs. J Vet Intern Med 2012;26:334–40.

90. Moore SA, Muñana KR, Papich JA, et al. Levetiracetam pharmacokinetics in healthy dogs following oral administration of single and multiple doses. Am J Vet Res 2010;71:337–41.

91. Moore SA, Muñana KR, Papich JA, et al. The pharmacokinetics of levetiracetam in healthy dogs concurrently receiving phenobarbital. J Vet Pharmacol Ther 2011;34(1):31–4.

92. Von Klopmann T, Rambeck B, Tipold A. Prospective study of zonisamide therapy for refractory idiopathic epilepsy in dogs. J Small Anim Pract 2007;48: 134–8.

93. Dewey CW, Guiliano R, Boothe DM, et al. Zonisamide therapy for refractory idiopathic epilepsy in dogs. J Am Anim Hosp Assoc 2004;40:285–91.

94. Chung JY, Hwang CY, Chae JS, et al. Zonisamide monotherapy for idiopathic epilepsy in dogs. N Z Vet J 2012;60(6):357–9.

95. Miller ML, Center SA, Randolph JF, et al. Apparent acute idiosyncratic hepatic necrosis associated with zonisamide administration in a dog. J Vet Intern Med 2011;25:1156–60.

96. Schwartz M, Muñana KR, Olby NJ. Possible drug-induced hepatopathy in a dog receiving zonisamide monotherapy for treatment of cryptogenic epilepsy. J Vet Med Sci 2011;73(11):1505–8.

97. Cook AK, Allen AK, Espinosa D, et al. Renal tubular acidosis associated with zonisamide therapy in a dog. J Vet Intern Med 2011;25:1454–7.

98. Dewey CW, Cerda-Gonzalez S, Levine JM, et al. Pregabalin as an adjunct to phenobarbital, potassium bromide, or a combination of phenobarbital and potassium bromide for treatment of dogs with suspected idiopathic epilepsy. J Am Vet Med Assoc 2009;235:1442–9.
99. Platt SR, Adams V, Garosi LS, et al. Treatment with gabapentin of 11 dogs with refractory idiopathic epilepsy. Vet Rec 2006;159:881–4.
100. Siao KT, Pypendop BH, Ilkiw JE. Pharmacokinetics of gabapentin in cats. Am J Vet Res 2010;71(7):817–21.
101. Cautela MA, Dewey CW, Schwark WS, et al. Pharmokinetics of oral pregabalin in cats after single dose administration. In Proceedings ACVIM Forum. Anaheim (CA): 2010. p. 739.
102. Ruehlmann D, Podell M, March P. Treatment of partial seizures and seizure-like activity with felbamate in SUL dogs. J Small Anim Pract 2001;42:403–8.
103. Read MR. Midazolam. Compendium 2002;24:774–7.
104. Tobias KM, Marioni-Henry K, Wagner R. A retrospective study on the use of acepromazine maleate in dogs with seizures. J Am Anim Hosp Assoc 2006; 42:283–9.
105. Levitski RE, Trepanier LA. Effect of timing of blood collection on serum phenobarbital concentrations in dogs with epilepsy. J Am Vet Med Assoc 2000;217: 200–4.

Canine Pediatric Dentistry

Amy J. Fulton, DVM[a,b], Nadine Fiani, BVSc[c],
Frank J.M. Verstraete, DrMedVet, MMedVet[d],*

KEYWORDS

- Canine pediatric dentistry • Pedodontics • Veterinary dentistry • Dogs
- Deciduous dentition

KEY POINTS

- Every practitioner should be comfortable with normal dental anatomy in puppies and young adult dogs.
- The first puppy examination should include a comprehensive oral examination, with special attention paid to the orthodontic evaluation as well as evaluation of any developmental defects, including cleft lips and palates.
- Several developmental anomalies can affect the teeth, such as enamel hypoplasia, and persistent deciduous teeth that may or may not have a clinical impact on the dog.
- Deciduous teeth and immature adult teeth are prone to fracture and can rapidly result in endodontic disease.
- Certain tumor types can occur in young patients, and awareness is key in early recognition of these diseases.

The oral examination is an important part of the physical examination of every patient. In neonate and adolescent dogs, it is important to inspect the oral cavity for congenital and acquired dental and oral pathology. This article reviews the more common pediatric and juvenile dental anomalies that affect dogs in order to provide a resource for the basic understanding of the oral cavity in these patients.

NORMAL DECIDUOUS DENTITION

The first puppy examination typically occurs at approximately 8 weeks of age. At this age, the deciduous dentition should be fully erupted (**Table 1**).[1,2] Each quadrant should have 3 deciduous incisor, 1 deciduous canine, and 3 deciduous premolar

The authors have no financial disclosures to acknowledge.
[a] Dentistry and Oral Surgery Service, William R. Pritchard Veterinary Medical Teaching Hospital Small Animal Clinic, School of Veterinary Medicine, University of California-Davis, One Shields Avenue, Davis, CA 95616, USA; [b] Cordova Veterinary Hospital, 2939 Mather Field Road, Rancho Cordova, CA 95670, USA; [c] Small Animal Specialist Hospital, 1 Richardson Place, North Ryde, New South Wales, Sydney 2113, Australia; [d] Department of Surgical and Radiological Sciences, School of Veterinary Medicine, University of California-Davis, One Shields Avenue, Davis, CA 95616, USA
* Corresponding author.
E-mail address: fjverstraete@ucdavis.edu

Table 1
Eruption times for teeth in dogs

	Deciduous Eruption Times (wk)	Permanent Eruption Times (mo)
Incisor teeth	3–4	3–4
Canine teeth	3	3–4
Premolar teeth	4–12	4–6
Molar teeth	N/A	5–7

teeth. There are no deciduous precursors of the first premolar or of the molar teeth. In respect to appearance, the incisor and canine teeth are smaller, slimmer, and sharper than their permanent successors, and the deciduous premolar teeth appear as diminutive versions of the permanent teeth that erupt behind them. For instance, the deciduous fourth premolar tooth looks like a smaller version of the permanent first molar tooth (**Fig. 1**).[1,3] The roots of deciduous premolar teeth also tend to diverge compared with their permanent successor.

At approximately 12 weeks of age, it is possible to see mixed dentition present, where both permanent and deciduous teeth have erupted (see **Table 1**).[1,3] If a deciduous tooth is congenitally absent, then the successional permanent tooth will also be absent, a point that is easy to confirm with a dental radiograph.[1] Teeth can be named by their anatomic location. Alternatively, dental numbering systems, such as the triadan system,[4] have frequently been used in veterinary medicine to give each tooth a 3-digit number, where each tooth is numbered first by quadrant, then anatomy. For example, the right maxilla, in the 100-quadrant, results in the maxillary right canine tooth labeled as 104. The left maxilla represents the 200-quadrant, the left mandible the 300-quadrant, and the right mandible the 400-quadrant. The deciduous teeth then follow suit, labeled as 500, 600, 700, or 800 for the right maxilla, left maxilla, left mandible, and right mandible, respectively.[4,5]

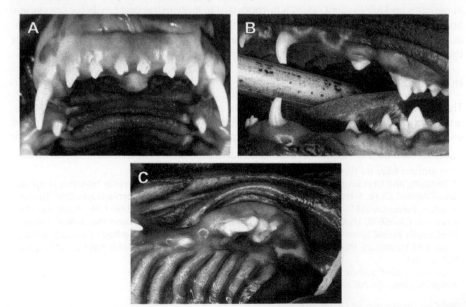

Fig. 1. Normal deciduous dentition in a 2-month-old dog: (*A*) maxillary incisor and canine teeth; (*B*) mandibular and maxillary canine and premolar teeth; (*C*) maxillary premolar teeth.

DEVELOPMENTAL ANOMALIES IN PUPPIES

Developmental anomalies of the maxillofacial structures that should be assessed in neonatal dogs include microglossia, ankyloglossia, and cleft lip or palate.

Microglossia and Ankyloglossia

Microglossia and ankyloglossia are rare genetic disorders that have been described as occurring in miniature schnauzers and Anatolian shepherds, respectively.[6-8] Microglossia is an exceedingly rare syndrome in which there is hypoplastic development of the tongue. This syndrome, which is typically fatal in dogs, has been reported in humans often in conjunction with limb deformities, although only 50 cases have been identified to date.[9] Ankyloglossia, also known as tongue-tie, is a congenital oral anomaly that may decrease mobility of the tongue and is caused by an unusually short, thick lingual frenulum. It may not require intervention in dogs until patients are older, unless they are unable to suckle normally.[8]

Cleft Lip and Cleft Palate

Congenital clefts occur sporadically and can involve the primary or secondary palate. They can occur spontaneously or can be induced secondary to certain drugs or other events that occur during fetal development.[10]

In normal palate development, neural crest cells that form the embryonic structures of the face and head migrate from laterally developing processes to fuse at the midline.[11] Any failure of these structures to migrate or to fuse leads to cleft formation.[10] The primary palate forms from the fusion of the nasal prominences and forms the lip and incisive bone. If the nasal prominences fail to form correctly, then a cleft lip or harelip develops (**Fig. 2**),[12-14] which can be unilateral or bilateral and often are asymptomatic. If the cleft involves the alveolar process of the incisive bone, there may be clinical signs associated with communication with the nasal cavity. Otherwise, closure of a cleft lip may be unnecessary or may be delayed until a patient is full-grown.

In humans, cleft lips are associated with cleft palates approximately 70% of the time.[12] Cleft palates involve the structures of the secondary palate, which separates

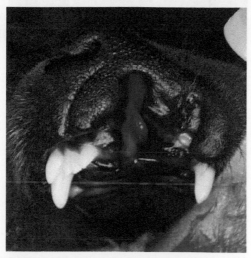

Fig. 2. A cleft of the primary palate, lip, and nostril in a 6-month-old dog. This cleft involved an oronasal communication at the level of the left maxillary second and third incisor teeth.

the oral and nasal cavities. Normal palate development results from the fusion of the maxillary processes, resulting in the formation of the hard and soft palate.[15] A defect in development may lead to a cleft in the hard palate caudal to the incisive bone, in the soft palate, or in both (**Fig. 3**). Congenital clefts of the hard palate are often midline, but soft palate clefts can be unilateral, bilateral, or on midline.[16,17] Also, patients with cleft palates often have other congenital abnormalities, including middle ear pathology, which can have a significant impact on the long-term prognosis for a puppy.[18,19]

Once diagnosed, a challenge in treating cleft palate patients is keeping patients healthy until they are of an age when surgery has the best chance of success, making supportive care and surgery a costly and time-intensive process. In cases of extensive secondary clefts, euthanasia may be the most appropriate option and should be recommended at the time the cleft is first noted. In addition, breeders should be advised of the implications of the genetic etiology of clefts on future breeding attempts.[10]

Repair of a cleft palate or lip is beyond the scope of this article and is discussed elsewhere.[10,14,16,20–23] Surgery should not be attempted by a casual operator because of the difficulty of surgery and high rate of complications. In all cases, surgery should be delayed as long as possible, because attempts to surgically repair a cleft prior to 3 or 4 months of age are unlikely to be successful and decrease future chance of success.[10,24–26] In children, attempts to repair clefts prior to 5 years of age was associated with facial growth deficiencies, similar to findings in research animals.[10] It has been stated by other investigators that the defect can become proportionally larger after 6 to 8 weeks of age.[2] A recent study identified a spontaneously occurring cleft palate in 15% to 20% of old Spanish pointers.[26] In measuring growth of these puppies with cleft palates, the investigators found that the cleft edges approach each other until 12 weeks of age, then separate significantly until 20 weeks of age, before they again

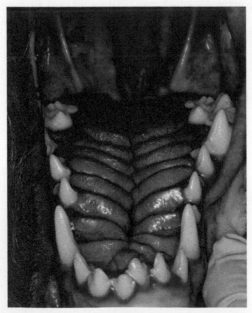

Fig. 3. Cleft of the secondary palate in a 5-month-old dog, involving the entire length of the hard and soft palate, in addition to a skeletal malocclusion of the maxillary incisor teeth.

approach one another.[26] This phenomenon has also been seen in other breeds of dogs with clefts[27] and is one of several good reasons to wait until a dog is at least 3 to 6 months old before any attempt at repair is made.

DELAYED ERUPTION OF TEETH

After examining the skeletal anatomy, the dentition of every puppy should be examined closely. Occasionally, deciduous or permanent teeth may fail to erupt. By 8 weeks of age, all deciduous teeth should be in their correct position, and by 6 months of age, all permanent teeth should be erupted. If a tooth is absent on oral examination, then dental radiographs should be obtained to confirm its absence or to document the presence of an unerupted or retained tooth.[2] If a tooth is impacted, implying that it is lying in abnormal position or has a physical impedance to its eruption, the tooth should be extracted. If a tooth is in a normal position and only covered by gingiva, then an operculectomy can be performed to provide a pathway of minimal resistance through which the tooth can erupt (**Fig. 4**).[28]

PERSISTENT DECIDUOUS TEETH

In certain cases, deciduous teeth may fail to exfoliate. The forces that guide resorption of the deciduous tooth root and exfoliation are tied to the forces of eruption of the secondary tooth.[3] The exact mechanisms by which this occurs, however, have not been elucidated. The deciduous tooth and its permanent counterpart should never be present in the oral cavity at same time (**Fig. 5**). If this occurs, the deciduous tooth is considered persistent and is likely to interfere with the normal eruption pathway of the permanent tooth; it is most commonly seen with the canine and incisor teeth, especially in toy breeds.[2] A strong genetic basis for this condition has been suggested although a multifactorial etiology cannot be excluded.[23] Persistent deciduous teeth cause crowding and alter the gingival contour, predisposing the area to periodontal disease as plaque and débris accumulate between the deciduous and permanent teeth.[2,23]

Persistent deciduous teeth should be extracted as early as possible in order to avoid malpositioned teeth and crowding. Even with early extraction, however, permanent teeth often continue to erupt in an abnormal position, and may require further orthodontic treatment after they are fully erupted.[2] If there is no permanent successor to a persistent deciduous tooth, and it is otherwise periodontally and endodontically healthy, then the tooth can remain as a functional tooth without interference.

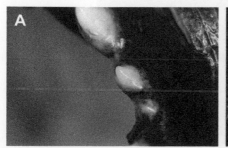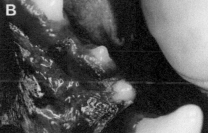

Fig. 4. (*A*) An unerupted right mandibular first premolar tooth in a 4-year-old dog; there is a thin layer of intact gingiva overlying the tooth. (*B*) The same patient after operculectomy has been performed to allow the tooth to completely erupt.

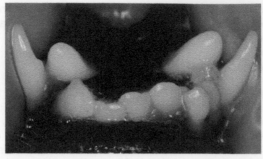

Fig. 5. Persistent deciduous mandibular canine teeth in a 9-month-old dog, with resultant linguoversion of the mandibular canine teeth that have only partially erupted. Note the increased food debris accumulating between the deciduous and adult canine teeth, along with the disruption of the normal gingival margin.

ENDODONTAL DISEASE IN DECIDUOUS TEETH

Deciduous teeth in general are thinner and more delicate compared with their permanent counterparts, making deciduous teeth especially subject to wear or fracture that results in pulp exposure (**Fig. 6**).[23] If left in place, the most likely sequelae include periapical lesion, osteomyelitis, and damage to the underlying developing permanent tooth. Regardless of intervention, the underlying permanent tooth may be damaged by the trauma that resulted in the deciduous tooth's injury. In the absence of a complicated crown fracture, pulp necrosis may also be evidenced by gray-tan crown discoloration. Endodontically diseased deciduous teeth should, in all cases, be extracted as soon after diagnosis as is reasonably possible.

EXODONTICS OF DECIDUOUS TEETH

The extraction of deciduous teeth should be performed with great care. These teeth are long, thin, and fragile and without careful flap design and extraction technique significant trauma to the developing permanent tooth can occur. If a tooth does fracture during removal, all efforts to carefully extract the root tip is crucial, because roots left behind can impede eruption of the permanent tooth. When considering extracting a deciduous tooth, it is essential to take preoperative dental radiographs to determine

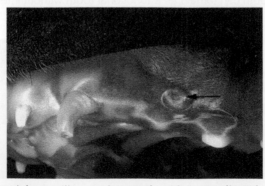

Fig. 6. A deciduous right maxillary canine tooth with a complicated crown fracture and discoloration. There is also a parulis (*arrow*) at the mucogingival junction, consistent with a periapical abscess.

the shape and location of the root and to document the presence and location of the developing permanent tooth.[2] Permanent incisor teeth erupt palatally or lingually to the deciduous incisor teeth, whereas permanent maxillary canine teeth erupt mesial to the deciduous tooth. The permanent mandibular canine teeth erupt mesially and lingually to the deciduous teeth.

NORMAL OCCLUSION

Even at 8 weeks of age, the deciduous teeth should be present and in appropriate occlusion, with normal interdigitation of teeth, integrity of the dental arches, and functioning of the temporomandibular joints (TMJs). The incisal margin of the mandibular incisor teeth should occlude against the cingulum, or enamel ridge, on the palatal aspect of the maxillary incisor teeth, forming a scissor bite. The mandibular canine tooth should be centered between the maxillary canine and maxillary third incisor, without touching either of these teeth. The tips of the crowns of the mandibular premolar teeth should fit in the interdental spaces of the maxillary premolar teeth, with each mandibular premolar tooth mesial to its maxillary premolar counterpart. Finally, the palatal surface of the deciduous maxillary third premolar should overlap the buccal surface of the mesial cusp of the deciduous mandibular fourth premolar tooth, and the occlusal surface present on the distal part of the deciduous mandibular fourth premolar tooth occludes with the occlusal surface of the deciduous maxillary fourth premolar tooth. In the adult occlusion, the permanent carnassial teeth, which are the maxillary fourth premolar and mandibular first molar teeth, occlude in the same manner as the deciduous maxillary third premolar and deciduous mandibular fourth premolar teeth do in puppies.[1] In this way, the deciduous occlusion reflects that of the adult. Occasionally, the upper and lower jaws may develop asynchronously, leading to a transitory mild malocclusion that is self-correcting.[1,2] If there are any skeletal or dental malocclusions noted on the first puppy examination at 8 weeks of age, however, then the adult dog will most likely exhibit the same malocclusion as their permanent teeth erupt.

MALOCCLUSIONS

Malocclusions are defined as an abnormal relationship between the teeth, jaws, and/ or the TMJ. Any deviation from the normal relationship is considered a malocclusion. Abnormal occlusions can be broadly divided into those of skeletal origin and those of dental origin. Skeletal malocclusions occur as a result of an abnormality in the morphology of the skull. Typically these are thought of as genetic defects, although they can also occur secondary to trauma to the developing maxillofacial structures. A dental malocclusion, alternatively, can be recognized when the skull morphology is normal and symmetric but 1 or more teeth are in an abnormal position.[1] Facial asymmetry, or an abnormal canine or premolar and molar occlusion, is typical of skeletal malocclusions, whereas abnormal incisor occlusion or individual malpositioned teeth are more common in dental malocclusions.

Malocclusions can also be classified on the basis of the relationship of the maxilla and mandible. In humans, the Angle classification is based on the relationship of the maxillary and mandibular first molar teeth.[29,30] Because this classification does not relate well to the carnivore dentition, the correct occlusion is based on the archetypal dog interdental and interarch relationships of the teeth. Following this principle, a neutrocclusion (class 1 malocclusion) can be defined as a normal rostral-caudal relationship of the maxillary and mandibular dental arches with malposition of 1 or more individual teeth. A mandibular distocclusion (class 2 malocclusion) is defined as an abnormal rostral-caudal relationship between the dental arches in which the mandibular arch occludes caudal to its normal position relative to the maxillary arch. A mandibular mesiocclusion (class 3 malocclusion) is defined as an abnormal rostral-caudal relationship between the dental arches in which the mandibular arch occludes rostral to its normal position relative to the maxillary arch.[5]

COMMONLY OBSERVED MALOCCLUSIONS

A rostral crossbite, one type of class 1 malocclusion, refers to a reverse relationship of the incisor teeth while the rest of the occlusion remains normal.[1] Often this affects all 6 incisor teeth, although only a few may be involved, and results in the maxillary incisors occluding lingually to the mandibular incisor teeth. This deviation of the incisor teeth is often due to palatoversion of the maxillary incisor teeth. A less severe form may lead to a level bite, where the incisor teeth meet end on, leading to attrition or wear of the incisor teeth over time.

Rostroversion of the maxillary canine tooth is another class 1 malocclusion where 1 or both maxillary canine teeth are deviated rostrally.[31–34] It is an abnormality encountered most commonly in Shetland sheepdogs and is sometimes referred to as lance or spear canine (**Fig. 7**).[35] The abnormal location of the tooth can be the result of persistent deciduous canines altering the eruption pathway. Possible complications arising from this malocclusion include crowding of the persistent deciduous canine and permanent maxillary canine teeth, a secondary buccoversion of the mandibular canine due to the maxillary canine impeding normal eruption, with resulting entrapment of the upper lip between the malpositioned canine teeth, leading to traumatic ulceration.

One of the most common malocclusions leading to trauma to the hard palate is a class 1 dental malocclusion, termed linguoversion of the mandibular canine teeth.[32,35] In this malocclusion, the teeth occlude lingually to their maxillary counterparts,

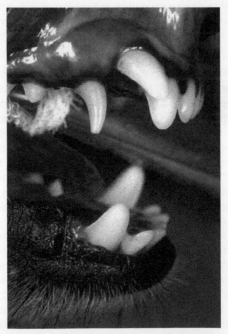

Fig. 7. A 7-month-old dog with a persistent deciduous canine tooth, resulting in rostroversion of the maxillary canine tooth.

causing trauma to the hard palate or the periodontium of the maxillary canine teeth. The cause is often delayed exfoliation of the deciduous mandibular canine teeth, forcing the permanent canine teeth to erupt lingually. Regardless of the cause, early treatment of both deciduous and permanent teeth should be considered to avoid ulceration of the hard palate and oronasal fistula formation.

Maxillary prognathism, mandibular brachygnathism, overshot, mandibular distocclusion, and class 2 malocclusion are all names that describe a mandible that is comparatively shorter than the maxilla.[5,29] This occlusion may be asymptomatic or can result in trauma to the hard palate by the mandibular canines or incisors depending on the degree of brachygnathism. The most severe form of mandibular brachygnathia is mandibular micrognathia, where the entire mandible is abnormally short and narrow (**Fig. 8**).[30] In these cases, the premolar and molar teeth are crowded, and the mandibular incisor and canine teeth can occlude several millimeters palatal to the maxillary teeth.

Class 3 malocclusions, where the maxilla is shorter than the mandible, is considered a breed standard in brachycephalic breeds. Colloquially, it is often referred to as an underbite or an undershot jaw. In dogs with this malocclusion, the mandibular canine and incisor teeth occlude buccally to the maxillary canine and incisor teeth. In most cases, this is actually due to a relative maxillary brachygnathism, in which the maxilla is underdeveloped. Although this may lead to crowding and rotation of the maxillary premolar teeth, intervention may not be necessary. Occasionally, however, there may be trauma to the soft tissues of the mandible and tongue that necessitates intervention.

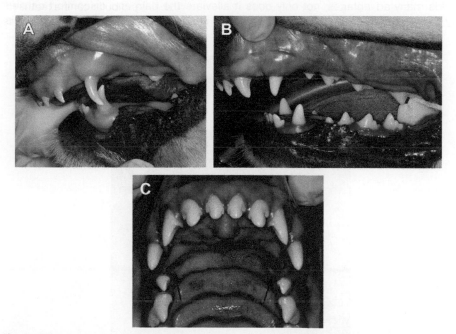

Fig. 8. (*A*) A 3-month-old puppy demonstrating a significantly underdeveloped mandible, known as mandibular micrognathia. The mandibular incisor teeth occlude several millimeters palatal to the maxillary incisor teeth. (*B*) The same patient at 6 months of age after the permanent dentition has fully-erupted. (*C*) The mandibular canine teeth have traumatized the hard palate leading to ulceration (*arrows*).

Wry bite is a lay term indicating facial asymmetry that has led to a skeletal malocclusion. It is a nonspecific term that should be replaced if possible with more descriptive terminology of the pathology.[5] For instance, there may be a mandibular-maxillary asymmetry in a dorsoventral direction (**Fig. 9**), which may lead to an open bite or to palatal trauma by the mandibular canine teeth that can have an impact on a patient's quality of life. As with other skeletal malocclusions, a wry bite may be of traumatic origin or due to a skeletal malformation.

TREATMENT OF MALOCCLUSIONS

In any case of a puppy diagnosed with a traumatic occlusion, where the deciduous teeth are causing trauma to the soft tissues of the mouth, interceptive orthodontics should be considered the most appropriate option for the deciduous dentition. By removing the deciduous tooth there is potential for an animal to achieve its full growth potential, by relieving any possible dental interlock that may be preventing mandibular growth.[2] Even if the malocclusion is too severe to expect a normal adult occlusion, it is important to minimize any soft tissue trauma, which, if affecting the hard palate, may result in oronasal fistula formation.

Correction of a malocclusion in adult patients has specific ethical considerations that should be considered and discussed, especially with regards to future breeding and showing attempts. If the occlusion is leading to pain and discomfort for a patient, several options for treatment are available.

Orthodontic correction of a malocclusion is a minimally invasive option and aims to move the teeth into a normal, or at least atraumatic, position. Orthodontic therapy holds many advantages; not only does it alleviate the pain and discomfort caused by the malocclusion but also it conserves the integrity of the tooth and jaw and it is

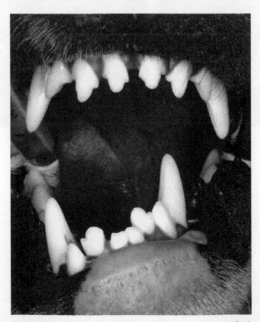

Fig. 9. Dorsoventral deviation of the mandible with crowding of the mandibular incisor teeth and linguoversion of the right mandibular canine tooth, consistent with a skeletal malocclusion, or wry bite.

the least invasive treatment option. Orthodontic treatment, however, also involves multiple anesthetic episodes to place, adjust, and remove any orthodontic device and can be uncomfortable for the patient while in place.

There are several options to orthodontically treat each malocclusion.[35] To treat linguoverted mandibular canine teeth, the placement of an orthodontic appliance, called an inclined plane, or bite plate, can be considered. Over several weeks, this appliance uses intermittent active force to move the mandibular canines buccally into an atraumatic position (**Fig. 10**). Another form of this therapy is to place crown extensions on the mandibular canines to help guide them into the appropriate position. In mild cases of mandibular canine linguoversion, ball therapy may be used. This therapy involves giving a patient a large rubber ball that the dog must carry in its mouth for several hours a day. The ball acts to push the mandibular canines buccally and into a correct occlusion (**Fig. 11**). These patients should be rechecked frequently, however, and, due to the possibility of failure, other treatment options should be discussed with the clients.

To orthodontically correct rostroverted maxillary canine teeth, an active force appliance can be used to pull the tooth distally into normal position, using buttons and a chain anchored on the maxillary fourth premolar and first molar teeth.

Each malocclusion has a unique presentation and requires a unique orthodontic treatment plan for successful correction of the malocclusion. Frequent follow-up examinations and adjustment of the orthodontic device as needed throughout treatment are key to successful orthodontic management of a malocclusion.

Crown height reduction and endodontic therapy is a good option for cases of traumatic occlusion, where a canine tooth is causing soft tissue trauma. This procedure involves amputating the crown of the canine tooth to remove the source of the trauma. In doing so, however, the pulp of the tooth is exposed, even when only removing a small portion of the crown. Endodontic therapy must be performed; otherwise, pulp necrosis and a periapical lesion ensue. Partial coronal pulpectomy or vital pulp therapy is a simple procedure that aims to conserve the vitality of the tooth while preventing infection of the pulp. Root canal treatment is another endodontic therapy option that can be performed if the tooth root has fully formed. Crown height reduction and partial coronal pulpectomy are often performed in cases of mandibular micrognathia or wry bite, where orthodontic treatment is not a realistic option.

Surgical extraction of any maloccluded tooth that is causing trauma is an acceptable option for certain clients and patients and as a salvage procedure. The main advantage of extraction is that once the tooth has been removed, no further procedures are needed. Alternatively, it is an invasive surgery, and if both mandibular canine teeth are removed, it results in considerable weakening of the rostral mandible.

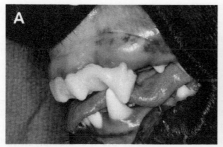
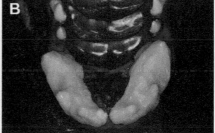

Fig. 10. Occlusal (*A*) and lateral (*B*) views of an inclined plane bite plate on the maxilla of a dog with linguoverted mandibular canine teeth.

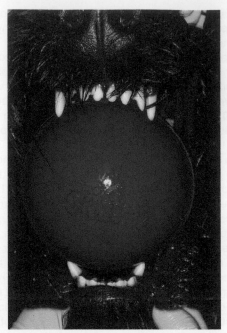

Fig. 11. In very mild cases of linguoverted canine teeth, a ball can be used to try to move the mandibular canine teeth buccally. The ball must fit snugly between the 2 canine teeth and the dog encouraged to play with the ball at least 2 to 3 hours per day.

Esthetically, a dog's tongue is not always contained within the oral cavity, which occasionally may result in moist dermatitis of the skin of the mandible in certain patients.

DEVELOPMENTAL ANOMALIES IN JUVENILE DOGS

At the 6-month check-up evaluation, all teeth should have erupted and it is at this point that abnormalities of the individual teeth may also be noted. A full oral examination should identify any persistent deciduous teeth or missing teeth, and with close inspection of the oral cavity during anesthesia for spay or neuter can be an efficient use of anesthetic time.

Dentigerous Cysts

If an unerupted tooth is left untreated, the enamel epithelium remains around the crown and can form a dentigerous cyst (**Fig. 12**). These odontogenic cysts enlarge over time, causing expansile destruction of the jaw and surrounding dentition.[36,37] The mandibular first premolar tooth is most commonly affected tooth and brachycephalic breeds are overrepresented.[37] Treatment is removal of the unerupted tooth and enucleation of the cyst lining.

Anatomic Anomalies

Several anatomic abnormalities may be encountered in canine patients. Some are considered incidental findings and are not of great clinical importance. Others may predispose patients to periodontal or endodontal disease or result in difficulty during extraction. Dental radiographs are indicated in cases of anatomic variation and prior to any extraction.

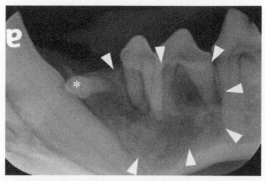

Fig. 12. Dental radiographs of the left rostral mandible demonstrating an impacted left mandibular first premolar tooth (*asterisk*) with a lucency surrounding the first, second, and third premolar tooth roots (*arrowheads*), representing a dentigerous cyst.

Gemination is a condition where a single tooth bud attempts to divide but results in the incomplete formation of 2 teeth.[23] Clinically, affected teeth usually have a longitudinal groove in the crown and a single root (**Fig. 13**), which should not be confused with fusion and concrescence.

Fusion and concrescence refer to the joining of 2 tooth buds to form a single structure.[23,38] The buds may be of 2 normally present teeth but may also occur between a normal tooth and a supernumerary tooth. Fusion may be complete or partial; however, the dentin is always confluent. When concrescence occurs, only the outermost cementum layer is continuous. This may also apply to the roots of a multirooted tooth, leading to a single root where there should be 2. This variation can be found in 23% of dogs and typically involves the premolar teeth.[39]

Both gemination and fusion may result in periodontitis due to an altered gingival contour.[23] Malocclusions and occlusal trauma can also occur with the altered anatomy.

Supernumerary roots may be present in some dogs. This anatomic variation is seen in 10.7% of dogs, most often resulting in a third root at the maxillary third premolar tooth. The presence of the extra root can result in an altered gingival contour and predispose to periodontitis.[38,39]

Dilaceration is another anatomic anomaly that may be observed in the root structure (**Fig. 14**). This is a sharp curve in the apical third of the root, commonly observed in the

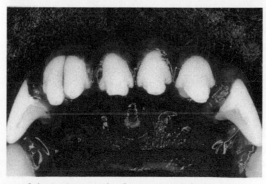

Fig. 13. Clinical image of the incisor teeth of a young adult dog, demonstrating bigeminy of the right second incisor teeth.

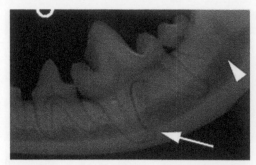

Fig. 14. Dental radiograph of the left caudal mandible demonstrating dilaceration, a marked deviation of the distal portion of the root, of the mesial root of the first molar tooth (*arrow*). Note that the second molar tooth also has fused roots (*arrowhead*).

mandibular premolar and molar teeth. It is not uncommon in dogs and has a reported prevalence of 3.5%.[39]

Occasionally the crown of a tooth may appear to have a folded or indented appearance. Known as dens invaginatus, this invagination of the enamel and dentin occurs during tooth development.[23,40] This abnormal fold in the hard tissues may result in external communication with the dental pulp and predispose to pulpitis, pulp necrosis, and eventually pulp infection.[23,40,41]

Enamel pearls are ectopic round masses of enamel that are frequently located at the cementoenamel junction.[23,42] These lesions can also predispose the tooth to periodontal disease by altering the gingival contour.

Abnormalities in Number of Teeth

Polydontia refers to an excessive or supernumerary number of permanent teeth. It can often result in crowding and create plaque retentive surfaces (**Fig. 15**). A well-recognized form of this condition is the mesiodens, which is a supernumerary maxillary incisor tooth found between the 2 first incisor teeth in brachycephalic breeds.[38] The reverse of polydontia is hypodontia, the congenital absence of 1 or more teeth. This condition is more common in the permanent dentition than the deciduous

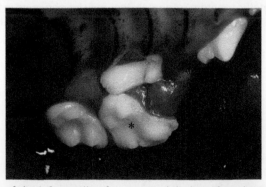

Fig. 15. Polydontia of the left maxilla of a young adult dog. There is a supernumerary first molar tooth inhibiting normal eruption of the fourth premolar tooth, leading to a palatoversion and incomplete eruption of this tooth (*asterisk*). (*From* Verstraete FJ. Oral pathology. In: Slatter DH, editor. Textbook of small animal surgery. vol. 2. 3rd edition. Philadelphia: Saunders; 2003. p. 2639; with permission.)

dentition.[23] If a deciduous tooth is missing, the corresponding permanent tooth is often absent also. In some cases, oligodontia, where only a few teeth are present, may be observed.[23] Rarely, anodontia, or complete congenital absence of teeth, which may involve both the deciduous and the permanent dentition, may occur.[23]

X-linked Hypohidrotic Ectodermal Dysplasia

Affected dogs have been shown to have many dental abnormalities.[43] More commonly affected breeds include Chinese crested and other hairless breeds. Dental abnormalities include hypodontia, oligodontia, conical-shaped crowns, reduced number of cusps, reduced number of roots, and dilacerated roots. The disorder may also be associated with malocclusion.

Localized Enamel Hypoplasia

Trauma or infection of a developing tooth may result in focal enamel hypoplasia.[23,44] Affected teeth are limited to 1 or a few adjacent teeth and are often referred to as Turner hypoplasia (**Fig. 16**).[45] Common conditions that may lead to trauma of the developing tooth are intrusive luxation and poorly performed extractions of the corresponding deciduous tooth. Endodontically compromised deciduous teeth that develop periapical disease may also lead to enamel hypoplasia of the permanent tooth or adjacent teeth.

Generalized Enamel Hypoplasia

In dogs, a well-documented cause of generalized enamel hypoplasia is infection with distemper virus during the period of tooth formation.[46,47] It typically affects many or all

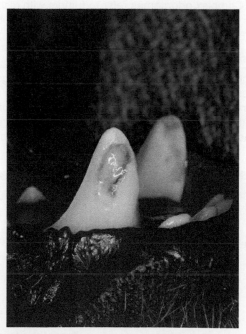

Fig. 16. Focal enamel hypoplasia affecting both mandibular canine teeth, likely as a result of trauma to the tooth bud during its development, such as a fracture or extraction of the deciduous mandibular canine tooth.

of the teeth, which, as a result, are predisposed to staining and calculus accumulation (**Fig. 17**).[48] The location of the hypoplastic areas may allow a clinical estimate of the time at which the infection occurred.[23] Extensive enamel hypoplasia may predispose the teeth to fracture or wear and lead to endodontic disease.

Intrinsic Tooth Discoloration

Systemic tetracycline administration during the age when the teeth are developing (2–6 months of age) can lead to incorporation of tetracycline into the enamel and dentin causing a permanent brown-yellow discoloration.[49–51] Tetracycline reacts with calcium forming a tetracycline-calcium orthophosphate complex. The pigmentation in the crown coincides with the part of the tooth developing at the time of drug administration.[49] The color can vary from lemon-yellow (demeclocycline and tetracycline) to yellow-gray and/or brownish (chlortetracycline and oxytetracycline).[52] Minocycline administration results in a blue-grayish pigmentation. Oxytetracycline gives the least discoloration. Doxycycline causes little dental discoloration.[52] The color can darken with exposure to light. Tetracyclines should not be administered to those pregnant or in the young patient with developing deciduous and permanent dentition. This form of staining is considered purely esthetic and no treatment is necessary.[52]

ORAL TUMORS IN JUVENILE DOGS
Odontomas

Odontomas are benign odontogenic tumors typically diagnosed in young dogs between 6 to 18 months of age. They are characterized by the presence of well-differentiated dental tissues, including enamel, dentin, and cementum.[53] When these tissues are organized into rudimentary toothlike structures, they are called compound odotomas (**Fig. 18**). Complex odontomas refer to tumors with disorderly organization of the conglomerate of dental tissues. Marginal excision and curettage to remove the abnormal tissue can be curative for these tumors.[53–55]

Canine Papillomatosis

The most common growth found in the oral cavity of immature dogs is oral papillomas. One study found these to represent as many as 16.4% of benign oral tumors.[56] Papillomas are wartlike raised nodules with frondlike projections of epithelium that can be found anywhere on the oral mucosa, tongue, palate, gingiva, and even pharynx. They can also occur on the nose, conjunctiva, and genital mucosa, although these are more

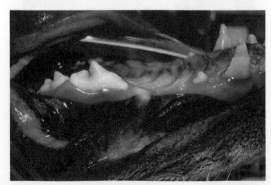

Fig. 17. Generalized enamel hypoplasia affecting all teeth at the same level in a dog that developed distemper viral infection at approximately 3 months of age.

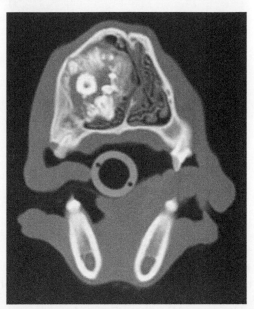

Fig. 18. CT image of a skull of a 1-year-old dog through the level of third premolar tooth demonstrating a mass expanding the right maxilla, causing expansion into the nasal cavity and deviation of the nasal septum. There are several tooth-shaped structures throughout the mass, consistent with a compound odontoma.

rare.[57] Caused by canine oral papillomavirus, this disease is transmissible and localized typically to the oral cavity.[58] The 55-nm DNA virus infects keratinocytes, causing them to transform and multiply, forming a papilloma.[59] This usually takes approximately 4 to 8 weeks from infection to papilloma formation, and the lesions typically spontaneously regress 4 to 8 weeks later.[57] Treatment of localized lesions is rarely indicated.

In certain individuals, however, the entire mouth can be covered in papillomas (**Fig. 19**), referred to as florid papillomatosis, and treatment may be indicated to help patients regain their normal ability to eat and drink.[60] Several therapies for florid papillomatosis have been described. The use of carbon dioxide–laser therapy to surgically remove papillomas has the advantage of coagulating the tumor as it is removed. Cryoablation, recombinant DNA vaccine, and autogenous vaccines derived from homogenized papilloma tissue have also been effective.[57,60,61]

Spontaneous regression of the tumor is related to a T-cell–mediated immune response, allowing the immune system to target and kill virus-infected cells.[59] Some efforts have been put into developing a preventative vaccine, with hopes of using it to help develop a similar human genital papillomavirus vaccine.[60]

Canine Oral Papillary Squamous Cell Carcinoma

Canine oral papillary squamous cell carcinoma (COPSCC) is a specific variant of oral squamous cell carcinoma that has been reported to occur in both young and old dogs.[54,56,62–64] COPSCC is an aggressive epithelial neoplasm that readily invades underlying bone (**Fig. 20**). If surgical excision of the tumor and involved bone and soft tissues is performed prior to any metastasis, a patient can be cured.[65,66] Radiation therapy for COPSCC has also been reported to have a good long-term prognosis in

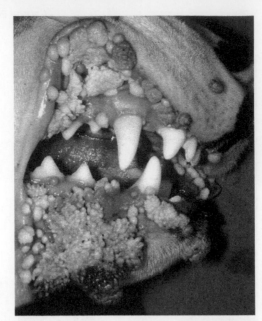

Fig. 19. A young pit bull terrier demonstrating florid papillomatosis of the tongue, buccal and alveolar mucosa, and skin. (*From* McEntee MC. Clinical behavior of nonodontogenic tumors. In: Verstraete FJ, Lommer MJ, editors. Oral and maxillofacial surgery in dogs and cats. 1st edition. Edinburgh (United Kingdom): Saunders; 2012. p. 398; with permission.)

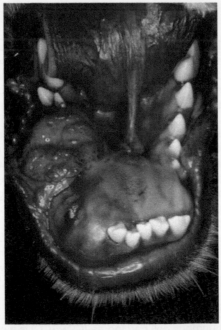

Fig. 20. COPSCC of the rostral mandible of a young dog, causing expansion of the rostral mandible, with deviation of the right mandibular fourth premolar and incisor teeth. There is an area of ulceration extending from the level of the first through third premolar teeth, which are absent in this dog. (*From* McEntee MC. Clinical behavior of nonodontogenic tumors. In: Verstraete FJ, Lommer MJ, editors. Oral and maxillofacial surgery in dogs and cats. 1st edition. Edinburgh (United Kingdom): Saunders; 2012. p. 390; with permission.)

dogs. Although infrequently reported, long-term side effects, such as osteoradionecrosis and secondary tumor formation at the site of radiation, are more likely given that patients have the potential to survive for a longer period of time than typical canine cancer patients.[67,68]

REFERENCES

1. Bezuidenhout AJ. Applied oral anatomy and histology. In: Slatter DH, editor. Textbook of small animal surgery, vol. 2, 3rd edition. Philadelphia: Saunders; 2003.
2. Hale FA. Juvenile veterinary dentistry. Vet Clin North Am Small Anim Pract 2005; 35(4):789–817.
3. Evans HE, de Lahunta A. Miller's anatomy of the dog. 4th edition. Philadelphia: Saunders; 2013.
4. Floyd MR. The modified Triadan system: nomenclature for veterinary dentistry. J Vet Dent 1991;8(4):18–9.
5. Nomeclature AVDC. Online. 2013. Available at: http://www.avdc.org/nomenclature.html. Accessed June 6, 2013.
6. Temizsoylu MD, Avki S. Complete ventral ankyloglossia in three related dogs. J Am Vet Med Assoc 2003;223(10):1443–5.
7. Wiggs RB, Lobprise HB, de Lahunta A. Microglossia in three littermate puppies. J Vet Dent 1994;11(4):129–33.
8. Karahan S, Kul BC. Ankyloglossia in dogs: a morphological and immunohistochemical study. Anat Histol Embryol 2009;38(2):118–21.
9. Voigt S, Park A, Scott A, et al. Microglossia in a newborn: a case report and review of the literature. Arch Otolaryngol Head Neck Surg 2012;138(8):759–61.
10. Kelly KM, Bardach J. Biologic basis of cleft palate and palatal surgery. In: Verstraete FJ, Lommer MJ, editors. Oral and maxillofacial surgery in dogs and cats. 1st edition. Edinburgh (United Kingdom): Saunders; 2012. p. 343–50.
11. Nanci A, Ten Cate AR. Ten Cate's oral histology: development, structure, and function. 8th edition. St Louis (MO): Elsevier; 2013.
12. Bender PL. Genetics of cleft lip and palate. J Pediatr Nurs 2000;15(4):242–9.
13. Howard GT Jr. The surgical repair and rehabilitation of the cleft palate and harelip patient. Am Surg 1953;19(5):441–53.
14. Arzi B, Verstraete FJ. Repair of a bifid nose combined with a cleft of the primary palate in a 1-year-old dog. Vet Surg 2011;40(7):865–9.
15. Miettinen PJ, Chin JR, Shum L, et al. Epidermal growth factor receptor function is necessary for normal craniofacial development and palate closure. Nat Genet 1999;22(1):69–73.
16. Warzee CC, Bellah JR, Richards D. Congenital unilateral cleft of the soft palate in six dogs. J Small Anim Pract 2001;42(7):338–40.
17. Gorlin RJ. Living history-biography: from oral pathology to craniofacial genetics. Am J Med Genet 1993;46(3):317–34.
18. White RN, Hawkins HL, Alemi VP, et al. Soft palate hypoplasia and concurrent middle ear pathology in six dogs. J Small Anim Pract 2009;50(7):364–72.
19. Gregory SP. Middle ear disease associated with congenital palatine defects in seven dogs and one cat. J Small Anim Pract 2000;41(9):398–401.
20. Marretta SM. Cleft palate repair techniques. In: Verstraete FJ, Lommer MJ, editors. Oral and maxillofacial surgery in dogs and cats. 1st edition. Edinburgh (United Kingdom): Saunders; 2012. p. 351–62.
21. Marretta SM, Grove TK, Grillo JF. Split palatal U-flap: a new technique for repair of caudal hard palate defects. J Vet Dent 1991;8(1):5–8.

22. Sager M, Nefen S. Use of buccal mucosal flaps for the correction of congenital soft palate defects in three dogs. Vet Surg 1998;27(4):358–63.

23. Verstraete FJ. Oral pathology. In: Slatter DH, editor. Textbook of small animal surgery, vol. 2, 3rd edition. Philadelphia: Saunders; 2003. p. 2638–51.

24. Bardach J, Kelly KM. Does interference with mucoperiosteum and palatal bone affect craniofacial growth? An experimental study in beagles. Plast Reconstr Surg 1990;86(6):1093–100.

25. Kremenak CR Jr, Kremenak CR Sr. Influence of occlusion on amount of jaw growth inhibition induced by palate surgery in beagles. J Dent Res 1970; 49(4):893.

26. Paradas-Lara I, Casado-Gomez I, Martin C, et al. Maxillary growth in a congenital cleft palate canine model for surgical research. J Craniomaxillofac Surg 2013. [Epub ahead of print]. http://dx.doi.org/10.1016/j.jcms.2013.01.032.

27. Kremenak CR Jr, Huffman WC, Olin WH. Growth of maxillae in dogs after palatal surgery. II. Cleft Palate J 1970;7:719–36.

28. Legendre L. Management of unerupted teeth. In: Verstraete FJ, Lommer MJ, editors. Oral and maxillofacial surgery in dogs and cats. 1st edition. Edingburgh (United Kingdom): Saunders; 2012. p. 525–9.

29. Hennet PR, Harvey CE, Emily PP. The Angle classification system of malocclusion: is it appropriate for use in veterinary dentistry? J Vet Dent 1992;9(3): 10–2.

30. Hennet PR, Harvey CE. Craniofacial development and growth in the dog. J Vet Dent 1992;9(2):11–8.

31. Hennet PR. Orthodontics. In: Slatter DH, editor. Textbook of small animal surgery, vol. 2, 3rd edition. Philadelphia: Saunders; 2003. p. 2686–95.

32. Hennet PR, Harvey CE. Diagnostic approach to malocclusions in dogs. J Vet Dent 1992;9(2):23–6.

33. Holmstrom SE, Fitch PF, Eisner ER. Orthodontics. In: Holmstrom SE, Frost P, Gammon RL, editors. Veterinary dental techniques: for the small animal practitioner. 3rd edition. Philadelphia: Saunders; 2004. p. 449–588.

34. Surgeon TW. Fundamentals of small animal orthodontics. Vet Clin North Am Small Anim Pract 2005;35(4):869–89.

35. Wiggs RB, Lobprise HB. Basics of orthodontics. In: Wiggs RB, Lobprise HB, editors. Veterinary dentistry: principles and practice. Philadelphia: Lippincott-Raven Publishers; 1997. p. 435–81.

36. Fulton A, Fiani N. Diagnostic imaging in veterinary dental practice. Dentigerous cyst with secondary infection. J Am Vet Med Assoc 2011;238(4):435–7.

37. Verstraete FJ, Zin BP, Kass PH, et al. Clinical signs and histologic findings in dogs with odontogenic cysts: 41 cases (1995-2010). J Am Vet Med Assoc 2011;239(11):1470–6.

38. Pavlica Z, Erjavec V, Petelin M. Teeth abnormalities in the dog. Acta Vet Brno 2001;70(1):65–72.

39. Verstraete FJ, Kass PH, Terpak CH. Diagnostic value of full-mouth radiography in dogs. Am J Vet Res 1998;59(6):686–91.

40. Duncan HL. Diagnostic imaging in veterinary dental practice. Dens invaginatus leading to arrested maturation of the right and left mandibular first molar teeth. J Am Vet Med Assoc 2010;237(11):1251–3.

41. Coffman CR, Visser CJ, Visser L. Endodontic treatment of dens invaginatus in a dog. J Vet Dent 2009;26(4):220–5.

42. Schneck GW. A case of enamel pearls in a dog. Vet Rec 1973;92(5):115–7.

43. Lewis JR, Reiter AM, Mauldin EA, et al. Dental abnormalities associated with X-linked hypohidrotic ectodermal dysplasia in dogs. Orthod Craniofac Res 2010;13(1):40–7.
44. Altun C, Cehreli ZC, Guven G, et al. Traumatic intrusion of primary teeth and its effects on the permanent successors: a clinical follow-up study. Oral Surg Oral Med Oral Pathol Oral Radiol Endod 2009;107(4):493–8.
45. Geetha Priya PR, John JB, Elango I. Turner's hypoplasia and non-vitality: a case report of sequelae in permanent tooth. Contemp Clin Dent 2010;1(4): 251–4.
46. Bittegeko SB, Arnbjerg J, Nkya R, et al. Multiple dental developmental abnormalities following canine distemper infection. J Am Anim Hosp Assoc 1995; 31(1):42–5.
47. Dubielzig RR, Higgins RJ, Krakowka S. Lesions of the enamel organ of developing dog teeth following experimental inoculation of gnotobiotic puppies with canine distemper virus. Vet Pathol 1981;18(5):684–9.
48. Fiani N, Arzi B. Diagnostic imaging in veterinary dental practice. J Am Vet Med Assoc 2009;235(3):271–3.
49. Bennett IC, Law DB. Incorporation of tetracycline in developing dog enamel and dentin. J Dent Res 1965;44:788–93.
50. Walton RE, O'Dell NL, Lake FT, et al. Internal bleaching of tetracycline-stained teeth in dogs. J Endod 1983;9(10):416–20.
51. Walton RE, O'Dell NL, Myers DL, et al. External bleaching of tetracycline stained teeth in dogs. J Endod 1982;8(12):536–42.
52. Verstraete FJ. Self-assessment color review of veterinary dentistry. London: Manson Publishing Ltd; 1999.
53. Chamberlain TP, Lommer MJ. Clinical behavior of odontogenic tumors. In: Verstraete FJ, Lommer MJ, editors. Oral and maxillofacial surgery in dogs and cats. 1st edition. Edinburgh (United Kingdom): Saunders; 2012. p. 403–10.
54. Withrow SJ, Vail DM. Withrow & MacEwen's small animal clinical oncology. 4th edition. St Louis (MO): Saunders Elsevier; 2007.
55. Regezi JA, Sciubba JJ, Jordan RC. Oral pathology: clinical pathologic correlations. 5th edition. St Louis (MO): Saunders/Elsevier; 2008.
56. McEntee MC. Clinical behavior of nonodontogenic tumors. In: Verstraete FJ, Lommer MJ, editors. Oral and maxillofacial surgery in dogs and cats. 1st edition. Edinburgh (United Kingdom): Saunders; 2012. p. 387–402.
57. Nicholls PK, Klaunberg BA, Moore RA, et al. Naturally occurring, nonregressing canine oral papillomavirus infection: host immunity, virus characterization, and experimental infection. Virology 1999;265(2):365–74.
58. Bredal WP, Thoresen SI, Rimstad E, et al. Diagnosis and clinical course of canine oral papillomavirus infection. J Small Anim Pract 1996;37(3):138–42.
59. Munday JS, Kiupel M. Papillomavirus-associated cutaneous neoplasia in mammals. Vet Pathol 2010;47(2):254–64.
60. Kuntsi-Vaattovaara H, Verstraete FJ, Newsome JT, et al. Resolution of persistent oral papillomatosis in a dog after treatment with a recombinant canine oral papillomavirus vaccine. Vet Comp Oncol 2003;1(1):57–63.
61. Jarrett WF, O'Neil BW, Gaukroger JM, et al. Studies on vaccination against papillomaviruses: a comparison of purified virus, tumour extract and transformed cells in prophylactic vaccination. Vet Rec 1990;126(18):449–52.
62. Nemec A, Murphy B, Kass PH, et al. Histological subtypes of oral non-tonsillar squamous cell carcinoma in dogs. J Comp Pathol 2012;147(2–3):111–20.

63. Soukup JW, Snyder CJ, Simmons BT, et al. Clinical, histologic, and computed tomographic features of oral papillary squamous cell carcinoma in dogs: 9 cases (2008-2011). J Vet Dent 2013;30(1):18–24.

64. Nemec A, Murphy BG, Jordan RC, et al. Oral papillary squamous cell carcinoma in dogs: 12 cases (1990-2012). J Comp Pathol, http://dx.doi.org/10.1016/j.jcpa.2013.07.007. [Epub ahead of print].

65. Stapleton BL, Barrus JM. Papillary squamous cell carcinoma in a young dog. J Vet Dent 1996;13(2):65–8.

66. Ogilvie GK, Sundberg JP, O'Banion MK, et al. Papillary squamous cell carcinoma in three young dogs. J Am Vet Med Assoc 1988;192(7):933–6.

67. McEntee MC, Page RL, Theon A, et al. Malignant tumor formation in dogs previously irradiated for acanthomatous epulis. Vet Radiol Ultrasound 2004;45(4):357–61.

68. Hosoya K, Poulson JM, Azuma C. Osteoradionecrosis and radiation induced bone tumors following orthovoltage radiation therapy in dogs. Vet Radiol Ultrasound 2008;49(2):189–95.

Successful Management Permitting Delayed Operative Revision of Cleft Palate in a Labrador Retriever

Autumn P. Davidson, DVM, MS[a,b,]*, Clare Gregory, DVM[b],
Patricia Dedrick, DVM[c]

KEYWORDS

- Congenital cleft palate • Labrador retriever
- Delayed operative revision of secondary cleft palate

KEY POINTS

- Affected neonates are diagnosed by visual inspection of the face and oral cavity.
- Methods to improve survival of puppies with congenital cleft palate (CP) are sought by clients; additionally, survival to reproductive age in congenitally affected dogs providing a research model for the human condition avoids the need for iatrogenic or teratogenically induced models.
- Feeding dry kibble and providing water from an overhead dispenser permits dogs with CP to attain adult size before reconstructive surgery, facilitating repair.

Congenital palate defects (CP) occur in dogs, with an incidence of up to 25%.[1] Secondary cleft palate (SCP) is a congenital oronasal fistula resulting in incomplete closure of the hard and soft palate. SCP occurs alone or in combination with primary cleft palate involving the lip and premaxilla. CP results from incomplete fusion of the palatine shelves, most critical at 25 to 28 days gestation, attributed to genetic (recessive or incompletely dominant polygenic inheritance), teratogenic (drugs, supplements), nutritional (folic acid deficiency), or infectious (viral) factors.[2]

Affected neonates are diagnosed by visual inspection of the face and oral cavity. Ineffective nursing/suckling results; these neonates fail to thrive, developing aspiration pneumonia and rhinitis. Feeding by orogastric tube is indicated until the puppy reaches a size permitting oral surgery, traditionally advised at 8 to 12 weeks of age.

[a] Veterinary Medical Teaching Hospital Small Animal Clinic, Department of Medicine and Epidemiology, School of Veterinary Medicine, University of California, 1 Shields Avenue, Davis, CA 95616, USA; [b] Pet Care Veterinary Hospital, East Campus, 2425 Mendocino Avenue, Santa Rosa, CA 95403, USA; [c] Dedrick Veterinary Services, 1515 Refugio Road, Santa Ynez, CA 93460, USA
* Corresponding author.
E-mail address: apdavidson@ucdavis.edu

Vet Clin Small Anim 44 (2014) 325–329
http://dx.doi.org/10.1016/j.cvsm.2013.11.002
0195-5616/14/$ – see front matter © 2014 Elsevier Inc. All rights reserved.

Palatoplasty in such young puppies remains difficult because of patient size and anticipated postoperative orofacial growth, often necessitating in multiple operations.[3] Esophagostomy and gastrostomy tube placement can facilitate feeding over time but require significant client commitment and can still result in aspiration. Palatal prostheses are problematic.[4,5]

Methods to improve survival of puppies with CP are sought by clients; survival to reproductive age in congenitally affected dogs providing a research model for the human condition avoids the need for iatrogenic or teratogenically induced models. This case report illustrates a successful method to manage nutrition in affected dogs until adult size is attained, facilitating surgical correction.

The diagnosis of SCP was made in a neonatal male Labrador retriever (**Fig. 1**). No history of drug or toxin exposure during the prepartum period was found. Upon diagnosis, feeding of the dam's colostrum for 24 hours, followed by artificial bitch milk replacer (Esbilac PetAg, Inc, Hampshire, IL) by intermittent orogastric tube was instituted. At 4 weeks of age, transition to a dry commercial pediatric dog food was made. The dry kibble diet was not soaked in water. Water was made available through an overhead ball point tube cap system (Lixit Animal Care Products, Napa, CA).

The dog thrived; the cleft monitored over time and partially closed spontaneously (**Figs. 2** and **3**). At 14 months of age (27 kg), surgical correction of the cleft palate was sought, because repeated episodes of foreign body entrapment above the palate had occurred. No episodes of aspiration pneumonia were noted.

Premedication with hydromorphone (Dilaudid [Abbott, Abbott Park, IL] 1 mg/mL) (0.1 mg/kg subcutaneously) was followed with propofol (PropoFlo [Abbott] 10 mg/mL) induction (6 mg/kg intravenously to effect) and maintenance anesthesia with sevoflurane (SevoFlo [Abbott])/O2. A sliding bipedicle mucoperiosteal flap repair was performed. Two incisions were made parallel to the dental arcade, creating 2 sliding mucoperiosteal flaps. The mucoperiosteum was elevated from the hard palate with

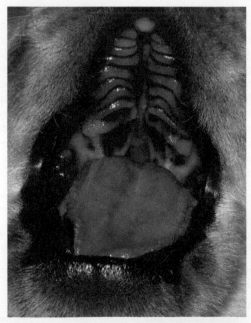

Fig. 1. Neonatal male Labrador retriever with a secondary cleft palate.

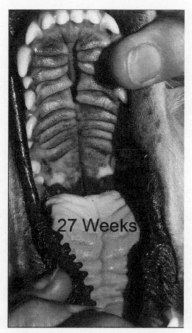

Fig. 2. Partially spontaneously closed secondary cleft palate at 27 weeks.

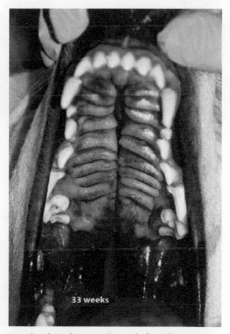

Fig. 3. Partially spontaneously closed secondary cleft palate at 33 weeks.

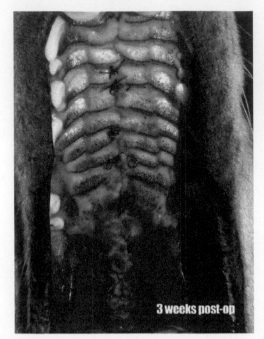

Fig. 4. Postoperative image of the healing secondary cleft palate revision at the time of suture removal.

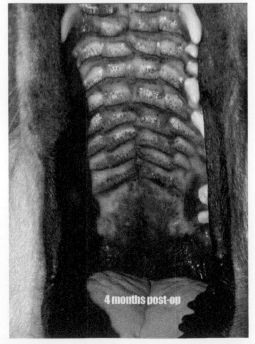

Fig. 5. Fully healed cleft palate at 4 months postoperatively.

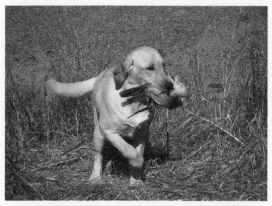

Fig. 6. The dog is normal more than a year post operatively without evidence of rhinitis or aspiration.

the major palatine artery. The nasal mucosa and mucoperiosteum were then opposed in a single layer over the defect in the hard palate, using 2-0 monocryl (Ethicon) in a simple interrupted pattern. The denuded hard palate near the dental arcades was left to heal by secondary intention. A fentanyl (Duragesic) 75 μg/h) transdermal patch was applied postoperatively. Clavamox 375 mg (300 mg amoxicillin 75 mg clavulanic acid) was administered for 10 days postoperatively at 375 mg twice daily by mouth.

A soft food diet was advised for 14 days with avoidance of chew toys. The site was healed at the time of suture removal in 14 days (**Fig. 4**). Subsequently, a dry dog food diet was successfully reinstituted. The dog is normal without rhinitis or aspiration 18 months postoperatively (**Figs. 5** and **6**). Feeding dry kibble and providing water from an overhead dispenser permits dogs with SCP to attain adult size before reconstructive surgery, facilitating repair.

REFERENCES

1. Richtsmeier JT, Sack GH, Grausz HM, et al. Cleft palate with autosomal recessive transmission in Brittany spaniels. Cleft Palate Craniofac J 1994;31(5):364–71.
2. Fossum TW. Surgery of the digestive system. In: Fossum TW, editor. Small animal surgery. 3rd edition. Philadelphia: Elsevier; 2002. p. 285–97.
3. Kirby BM. Oral flaps: principles, problems and complications of flaps for reconstruction of the oral cavity. Probl Vet Med 1990;2:494.
4. Martínez-Sanz E, Casado-Gómez I, Martín C, et al. A new technique for feeding dogs with a congenital cleft palate for surgical research. Lab Anim 2011;45(2): 70–80.
5. Kuipers von Lande RG, Worth AJ, Peckitt NS, et al. Rapid prototype modeling and customized titanium plate fabrication for correction of a persistent hard palate defect in a dog. J Am Vet Med Assoc 2012;240(11):1316–22.

Pediatric Feline Upper Respiratory Disease

Jane E. Sykes, PhD

KEYWORDS

- Feline herpesvirus-1 • Feline calicivirus • *Mycoplasma* • *Streptococcus* • *Chlamydia*
- Famciclovir

KEY POINTS

- Feline upper respiratory tract disease (URTD) is an important cause of morbidity and mortality in kittens, especially those held in population-dense and unhygienic conditions.
- Multiple bacterial and viral pathogens are involved and can cause similar clinical signs.
- Caution is required when interpreting the results of diagnostic tests for feline URTD pathogens because the presence of the pathogen does not always imply disease causation.
- Famciclovir or topical cidofovir are emerging as effective antiviral treatments for kittens with severe URTD that is caused by feline herpesvirus-1, but these drugs are not effective for other causes of feline URTD and indiscriminate use may result in drug resistance.
- Reducing stress and overcrowding in combination with vaccination and proper disinfection is likely to be the most effective means to prevent feline URTD in kittens housed in population-dense environments.

INTRODUCTION

Infectious feline upper respiratory tract disease (URTD) continues to be a widespread and important cause of morbidity and mortality in kittens, especially those held together in overcrowded or stressful conditions.[1] The clinical signs of disease vary considerably in severity and include lethargy, inappetence, sneezing, conjunctival hyperemia, serous to mucopurulent nasal and ocular discharges, hypersalivation, and in some cases respiratory distress caused by bronchopneumonia and death.

Multiple pathogens can contribute to URTD in kittens, and coinfections are common in overcrowded environments and contribute to increased disease severity. Worldwide, the most prevalent pathogens are feline herpesvirus-1 (FHV-1) and feline calicivirus (FCV). Mucopurulent discharges that develop in cats with these viral infections result from secondary bacterial infections with opportunistic pathogens, such as

Department of Medicine and Epidemiology, University of California, Davis, 2108 Tupper Hall, Davis, CA 95616, USA
E-mail address: jesykes@ucdavis.edu

Vet Clin Small Anim 44 (2014) 331–342
http://dx.doi.org/10.1016/j.cvsm.2013.10.005
0195-5616/14/$ – see front matter © 2014 Elsevier Inc. All rights reserved.

Streptococcus spp, *Staphylococcus* spp, *Pasteurella multocida*, and *Escherichia coli*. Primary bacterial causes of URTD disease in cats include *Bordetella bronchiseptica*, *Chlamydia felis*, and *Mycoplasma* spp. *Streptococcus canis* and *Streptococcus equi* subspecies *zooepidemicus* occasionally play a role as primary pathogens in shelter situations and catteries.

This article reviews the major causes of disease in kittens, and provides an update on treatment and prevention strategies.

FELINE HERPESVIRUS-1 INFECTION

Most cats are likely exposed to FHV-1 during their lifetime. The virus survives less than a day at room temperature and is readily inactivated by most disinfectants. As a result, transmission occurs primarily through close contact, although fomites are likely to be an important mode of transmission in crowded environments. FHV-1 has been detected using culture in 0% to 39% of cats with URTD, although when sensitive polymerase chain reaction (PCR) assays are used to detect FHV-1, infection prevalences close to 100% have been detected in some groups of cats with acute respiratory disease.[2] The prevalence of shedding by apparently healthy cats ranges from 0% to 10%, and most often has been lower than 2%.[1,3-9] Virtually all infected kittens develop latent infection after recovery, which primarily occurs in the trigeminal ganglia. Reactivation of shedding, with or without concurrent clinical signs of URTD, occurs in less than half of latently infected cats 4 to 12 days after stress.[10] Reactivation of shedding by queens during lactation is thought to be an important contributor to new kitten infections.

Clinical signs of FHV-1 infection in kittens vary considerably in severity, from intermittent sneezing and conjunctivitis to severe bronchopneumonia and death. Although FHV-1 prefers to replicate in the lower temperatures of the upper respiratory tract, systemic infection with viremia may be more likely to occur in neonates. Damage to the upper respiratory epithelium may be followed by osteolysis of the nasal turbinates and persistent or recurrent sinusitis and rhinitis. In kittens with physiologic ankyloblepharon (adhesion of the ciliary edges of the eyelids), ocular infection may lead to the accumulation of pus in the conjunctival sac (conjunctivitis neonatorum) (**Fig. 1**).

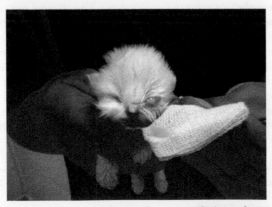

Fig. 1. Conjunctivitis neonatorum results in the accumulation of pus under the closed eyelids of neonatal kittens. Feline herpesvirus-1 is commonly implicated. (*From* Little SE. Pediatrics. In: Little SE, editor. The cat: clinical medicine and management. 1st edition. Philadelphia: Saunders; 2011. p. 1242; with permission.)

Symblepharon (adhesion of the conjunctiva to the cornea) can also occur and result in blindness (**Fig. 2**). Replication of FHV-1 in corneal epithelial cells[11] may be followed by the development of dendritic or geographic corneal ulceration and keratitis in some kittens. Occasionally, FHV-1 infection is associated with severe ulcerative and eosinophilic facial dermatitis (**Fig. 3**).

FELINE CALICIVIRUS INFECTION

Like FHV-1, FCV is a common cause of feline URTD, and accounts for 10% to more than 50% of cases. Genetically, isolates worldwide are a single, but highly diverse group. Infected cats can develop persistent infection of the oropharyngeal tissues (>1 month in duration) with shedding in the absence of obvious clinical signs. These cats are an important source of infection for other cats. In many cats, shedding terminates weeks to months after infection, but in a few cats, shedding continues for the duration of the cat's life. A single cat may be infected with multiple variants of FCV at the same time, each derived from the original infecting strain as a result of genetic mutation, drift, and selection pressures.[12] Because of this carrier state, as many as one in five healthy cats in some cat populations can be shedding FCV.[7] Survival of FCV in the environment has been demonstrated for up to 28 days, and the virus resists routine disinfection with quaternary ammonium compounds.[13] As a result, fomites are an important means of transmission.

The clinical signs of FCV infection are highly variable. Ulcerative glossitis and ulceration of the nasal planum, conjunctiva, and skin are suggestive of FCV infection, but not all cats with FCV infection have oral cavity involvement; for example, some cats only have ocular and/or nasal discharges (**Fig. 4**). Persistent infection with FCV has also been linked to chronic ulceroproliferative and lymphoplasmacytic stomatitis, which involves the mucosa lateral to the palatoglossal arches (caudal stomatitis), the alveolar mucosa in the premolar and molar area, and sometimes the buccal mucosa (alveolar/buccal mucositis), although this is more often described in young adult cats than in kittens.[14–16]

Highly virulent strains of FCV have been isolated from outbreaks of severe systemic febrile illness in cats in the United States and Europe known as virulent systemic

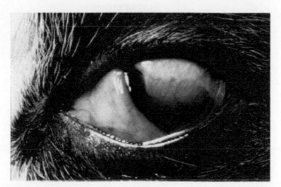

Fig. 2. Symblepharon in a cat following recovery from feline herpesvirus type 1 infection. Conjunctiva has adhered to the cornea dorsally (where it is visible as a thin white, vascular membrane) and the third eyelid conjunctiva has adhered to adjacent palpebral conjunctiva causing the third eyelid to remain partially protruded over the globe. (*From* Aroch I, Ofri R, Sutton GA. Ocular manifestations of systemic diseases. In: Maggs D, Miller P, Ofri R, editors. Slatter's Fundamentals of Veterinary Ophthalmology. 5th edition. Philadelphia: Saunders; 2012. p. 377; with permission.)

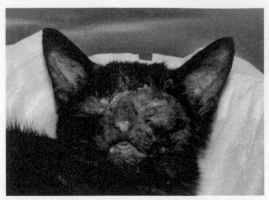

Fig. 3. Severe, erosive and exudative facial dermatitis associated with feline herpesvirus-1 infection in a 6-month-old female domestic shorthair cat. (*From* Gutzwiller ME. Use of interferon omega for skin diseases. In: August JR, editor. Consultations in feline internal medicine. vol. 6. Philadelphia: Saunders; 2010. p. 385; with permission.)

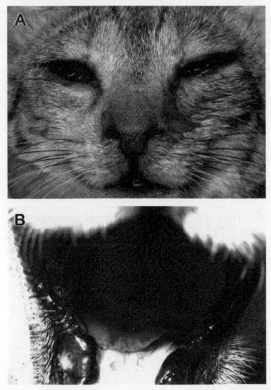

Fig. 4. Chemosis, mucopurulent ocular and nasal discharge (*A*), and lingual ulceration (*B*) in a 6-month-old intact male domestic medium hair cat with chronic nasal discharge and conjunctivitis. A conjunctival swab specimen tested positive with a PCR assay for FCV RNA and negative for FHV-1, *Chlamydia felis*, and *Mycoplasma* spp. (*Courtesy of* the UC Davis Veterinary Ophthalmology Service, with permission; and *From* Sykes JE. Feline respiratory viral infections. In: Sykes JE, editor. Canine and feline infectious diseases. 1st edition. Philadelphia: Saunders; 2013. p. 241, with permission.)

disease (VSD).[17-22] Clinical signs include anorexia, fever (often >105°F [40.6°C]), weight loss, oral and footpad ulceration, and nasal and/or ocular discharge. VSD strains infect not only epithelial cells of the upper respiratory tract and oral cavity, but also endothelial cells, hepatocytes, pneumocytes, and pancreatic acinar cells.[23] Distinctive clinical signs of VSD infection include cutaneous edema, alopecia, crusting, and ulceration. Edema occurs most commonly on the head and limbs but may become generalized, and crusting and ulceration are most prominent on the nose, lips, pinnae, periocularly, and on the distal limbs. Severe respiratory distress, sometimes caused by pulmonary edema or pleural effusion, develops in some cats. Involvement of the gastrointestinal tract, liver, and pancreas may also be associated with vomiting, icterus, and/or diarrhea. Cats also develop bleeding tendencies, which may occur as a result of vasculitis and disseminated intravascular coagulation, which can be manifested by petechial and ecchymotic hemorrhages, and rarely, epistaxis and hematochezia. In peracute infections, cats may die with few preceding signs apart from fever. Hospitalized shelter cats have been a source of infection in many outbreaks, and for each outbreak, the FCV strain involved differs, although recent research has identified common amino acid substitutions in the capsid protein gene that may distinguish VSD strains from those that are less pathogenic.[24] Otherwise healthy, adult, vaccinated cats are often most severely affected, but VSD has also been described in kittens. Outbreaks usually resolve within approximately 2 months once appropriate control measures have been instituted.

CHLAMYDIOSIS

Chlamydiae are obligately intracellular bacteria that primarily cause an acute to chronic or recurrent, follicular conjunctivitis in young adult cats. The main species infecting cats is C felis, but recently DNA that resembles that of the human pathogen Chlamydophila pneumoniae has been detected in ocular swabs from cats with conjunctivitis from Europe.[25]

Physical examination findings in cats with chlamydiosis include conjunctivitis, chemosis, serous to mucopurulent ocular discharge, and blepharospasm. Signs of nasal involvement, such as stertorous respiration, serous or mucopurulent nasal discharge, and sneezing, may accompany conjunctivitis. Chlamydiae may also play a role in other systemic and reproductive disorders in cats that remain poorly characterized.

Infection with C felis is most commonly detected in cats that are 2 to 12 months of age. Kittens less than 2 months of age may be protected by maternal antibody, although neonatal infections have been described. Chlamydial elementary bodies, the infectious form of the organism, survive only a few days in the environment at room temperature and are readily inactivated by most disinfectants, so transmission occurs primarily by direct contact. As a result, C felis infections are most commonly identified in multiple cat households, and especially those from breeding catteries. In cats from 218 European rescue shelters, breeding establishments, and private households, suboptimal hygiene was a risk factor for infection. C felis DNA is uncommonly detected in conjunctival swabs from healthy cats.[26] Coinfections with other respiratory pathogens, such as FHV-1 and FCV, are common and may contribute to increased severity of clinical signs.

BORDETELLOSIS

Bordetella spp are small, pleomorphic, gram-negative coccobacilli. The only Bordetella spp known to cause disease in dogs and cats is B bronchiseptica, but there are a large number of different strains of B bronchiseptica that vary in virulence and host specificity. Molecular typing efforts have shown that strains that infect dogs can be passed to cats and vice versa.[27–29] As for viral respiratory infections, bordetellosis is especially prevalent in cats in some shelter, pet store, and boarding facilities where large numbers of potentially stressed animals may have been in close contact with one another. Infections with *B bronchiseptica* frequently occur in concert with respiratory viral and/or *Mycoplasma* spp infections. *B bronchiseptica* can persist in the environment for at least 10 days and is capable of growth in natural water sources,[30] but is susceptible to most disinfectants provided they are used correctly. *B bronchiseptica* can be isolated from apparently healthy cats and cats with respiratory disease, but has been clearly associated with respiratory disease in cats. In one large European study that included 1748 cats from private multicat households, shelters, and breeding catteries, the larger the number of cats in the group, the greater the chance of detection of *B bronchiseptica*. In rescue shelters, increased seroprevalence was associated with poor hygiene.[1]

Clinical signs of bordetellosis in cats differ considerably in severity and may reflect such factors as bacterial strain, host immunity, and coinfections. Cats may show signs of sneezing and mucopurulent ocular and nasal discharge, but cough is uncommon.[31] Young kittens are more likely to show clinical signs than adults and may develop severe and life-threatening bronchopneumonia, with signs of tachypnea, cyanosis, and death.

MYCOPLASMA INFECTIONS

Mycoplasmas are fastidious bacteria that lack a cell wall and are found widely in association with mucous membranes of all mammalian species. The spectrum of mycoplasma species that infect dogs and cats is incompletely understood because precise species identification has been difficult. Because mycoplasmas are commonly isolated from the upper respiratory tract of healthy cats, their role in URTD has been difficult to determine. Stressors, such as overcrowding, concurrent respiratory viral infections, and unhygienic conditions, may also promote proliferation of mycoplasmas and their transmission between cats. Several studies have found an increased prevalence of mycoplasmas in cats with conjunctivitis or upper respiratory disease when compared with healthy cats.[26,32,33] Some mycoplasma species, such as *Mycoplasma felis*, may be more likely to cause disease than others. Clinical signs include nasal discharge and sneezing, serous to mucopurulent ocular discharge, conjunctival hyperemia, and possibly also keratitis.

STREPTOCOCCUS INFECTIONS

Organisms in the genus *Streptococcus* are gram-positive cocci that divide along a single axis, forming pairs and chains of organisms. Streptococci often invade tissues opportunistically when there is a breach in normal host barriers. Streptococci that infect cats range from commensal organisms of low virulence through to highly virulent organisms capable of causing severe disease manifestations and death. Neonatal bacteremia and sepsis can occur in kittens when organisms are transmitted from the vaginal tract during parturition. The organism may gain access to the systemic circulation by the umbilical vein. Purulent rhinosinusitis and pneumonia may occur in young cats in association with infections with other respiratory pathogens, such as respiratory viruses. Outbreaks of pneumonia, purulent rhinosinusitis, and meningoencephalitis caused by *S canis* and *S equi* subspecies *zooepidemicus* have occurred in cats housed in shelter environments.[34–37] As a result, *Streptococcus* spp should not always be dismissed as secondary invaders when isolated from outbreaks of URTD.

Isolation of the same organism from multiple affected cats in a cattery or shelter can add weight for their primary role in disease causation.

DIAGNOSIS

The cause of transmissible respiratory disease in kittens is not readily apparent based on clinical signs alone, because each pathogen produces a similar spectrum of signs. Although the presence of corneal ulceration raises suspicion for FHV-1 infection and ulcerative glossitis raises suspicion for FCV infection, mixed infections with respiratory viruses and bacteria occur commonly in crowded environments and complicate diagnosis. Given the widespread nature of disease in kittens and that mild to moderate clinical signs frequently resolve without treatment, specific diagnostic tests for feline upper respiratory tract pathogens are generally only applied when clinical signs are severe (such as when accompanied by pneumonia) or persistent (>7–10 days), or when multiple animals in a household are affected and information is required to aid treatment or control strategies. Assays that are widely available for diagnosis of feline upper respiratory tract infections include bacterial culture (for *Streptococcus* spp and bordetellosis) and PCR assays (for all pathogens discussed in this article). Cell culture for viruses (virus isolation) and chlamydiae are offered by some specialty diagnostic laboratories (eg, Animal Health Diagnostic Center at Cornell University) and has the potential to identify novel respiratory pathogens, or yield a diagnosis when PCR assays are negative. Cell culture for viruses should be considered to investigate outbreaks accompanied by clinical signs that are atypical, such as those accompanied by a high rate of kitten mortality. Serology for FCV has been of use for investigation of outbreaks that involved hypervirulent FCV strains.

Both positive and negative diagnostic test results for feline URTD pathogens must be interpreted with caution for the reasons shown in **Table 1**. PCR panels that include assays for multiple respiratory pathogens can be useful when applied to oropharyngeal or conjunctival swab specimens from multiple sick and healthy cats in a household to understand the range of pathogens present and their association with disease, and testing is also encouraged in individual cats if specific antiviral drug therapy is being considered. Topical anesthetics and fluorescein can reduce the sensitivity of PCR assays for human herpesviral infections, and so they should be avoided when

Table 1	
Considerations when interpreting diagnostic test results for upper respiratory tract pathogens in kittens	
Test Result	**Considerations**
Positive	Because virus can be shed by healthy cats, positive test results do not imply disease causation
	Positive test results can reflect recent vaccination with attenuated live vaccine organisms
	False-positive PCR test results can occur as a result of contamination of reactions in the laboratory or as a result of poor assay design
Negative	Some infected cats shed low numbers of organisms that are undetectable
	Poor PCR assay design can lead to false-negative results
	Degradation of nucleic acid during transport or inhibitors of PCR can lead to false-negative results
	Sequence variations in a pathogen's genome leads to false-negative PCR results

Abbreviation: PCR, polymerase chain reaction.

collecting conjunctival swab specimens.[38] Clean examination gloves should be worn for each cat tested and the swab should only touch the anatomic site to be tested.

Kittens that die with signs of URTD should be submitted for necropsy by a veterinary pathologist as soon as possible after death or euthanasia. Necropsy may allow identification of viral inclusions in respiratory tissues. Immunohistochemical stains, PCR assays, bacterial culture, or cell culture can be applied to increase the sensitivity for detection of respiratory pathogens in tissues obtained at necropsy (**Fig. 5**). The use of PCR and cell culture may provide optimum sensitivity for detection of viral infection when obtaining a diagnosis is of critical importance.

TREATMENT

Mild to moderate acute infections in neonatal stray and shelter kittens are widespread and many resolve over time without the need for antimicrobial treatment. Kittens with moderate to severe URTD that is accompanied by mucopurulent discharges may require supportive care consisting of fluid therapy, antimicrobial drugs for secondary bacterial infection, and enteral nutrition through the use of temporary feeding tubes. Because of its activity against *Bordetella* and mycoplasmas, doxycycline (10 mg/kg by mouth [PO] every 24 hours or 5 mg/kg PO every 12 hours) is recommended if antimicrobial treatment is deemed necessary. If chlamydiosis is suspected or confirmed, treatment for 4 weeks is recommended, and all cats in the household should be treated. Amoxicillin (12–20 mg/kg PO every 12 hours) is a reasonable second choice for treatment of secondary bacterial infections in cats with URTD, but does not have activity against mycoplasmas. Hospitalization and treatment with parenteral fluids, antimicrobial drugs, nebulization, and supplemental oxygen may be necessary for kittens that develop severe URTD and bronchopneumonia. Acute URTD generally resolves within 2 to 3 weeks with supportive care, but some cats experience frequent disease relapses and chronic complications, such as recurrent or persistent nasal discharge and keratitis.

The use of antiviral drugs could be considered for kittens with severe or persistent manifestations of FHV-1 infection (such as keratitis, severe conjunctivitis, and

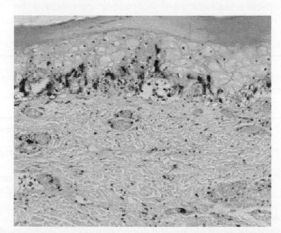

Fig. 5. Section of skin from a cat with virulent systemic feline calicivirus (FCV) infection. Strong anti-FCV immunoreactivity (*brown stain*) is observed within the basal layer of the epithelium and scattered in endothelial cells of the dermis. There is extensive epithelial necrosis. (*From* Foley JE. Calicivirus: spectrum of disease. In: August JR, editor. Consultations in feline internal medicine. vol. 5. Philadelphia: Saunders; 2010. p. 6; with permission.)

ulcerative facial dermatitis). Famciclovir (40–90 mg/kg PO every 8 hours) is the most potent and safe antiviral drug, and has been well tolerated when administered orally to kittens.[39] Treatment with famciclovir results in significant clinical improvement in cats with both acute and chronic herpesviral disease and decreased viral shedding.[40,41] Topical ophthalmic preparations that contain idoxuridine, trifluridine, vidarabine, and, to a lesser extent, acyclovir have been used to treat herpesviral keratitis, although the true efficacy of these drugs has not been extensively studied. Frequent topical application is required (five to six times daily), and prolonged use may cause corneal irritation or ulceration. Cidofovir (0.5% compounded solution in artificial tears administered twice daily) shows greater promise as a topical treatment and is active against FHV-1 in vitro and in experimentally infected cats.[42] The reader is referred to several recent reviews for more information on systemic and topical antiviral drugs for cats with FHV-1 infections.[39,43,44] Because antiviral drug-resistant strains of FHV-1 have been described, the use of such drugs as famciclovir should be reserved for cats with severe clinical signs that are suggestive of FHV-1 infection, and preferably in conjunction with molecular diagnostic testing to confirm the presence of FHV-1.

Human recombinant interferon-α and recombinant feline interferon-ω, which inhibit FHV-1 replication in vitro, have been administered parenterally, topically (for keratitis), and orally to cats with FHV-1 infection. In general, obvious clinical responses to treatment have not been uniformly observed, and controlled clinical trials that involve large numbers of cats are lacking. The amino acid lysine has shown efficacy for treatment of herpesviral conjunctivitis in cats when administered as tablets[45] and has reduced reactivated shedding by latently infected cats.[46] However, the efficacy of lysine has recently come into question after a lack of apparent activity in in vitro studies and lack of efficacy when administered to cats in shelters.[47] Finally, intranasal vaccines are currently being studied for their ability to treat cats with URTD (ie, as immunotherapeutics), with some promising preliminary results.[48]

PREVENTION

Prevention of URTD in kittens in cattery or shelter situations relies on minimizing stress and overcrowding, disinfection, quarantine, and vaccination. During the last 5 years, it has become increasingly apparent that measures to reduce stress and overcrowding can have a significant impact on reducing the incidence of URTD[49] and may be more important than quarantine. Cats should be housed singly, away from barking dogs, and given a place to retreat to or hide. The reader is referred to other resources for more information on reducing stress in shelter situations. Barriers between cats should be impermeable, and cats should be separated by at least 4 to 5 ft to prevent aerosol transmission. Disinfection should be performed using products active against FCV, such as potassium peroxymonosulfate (Trifectant, Virkon S), 1:32 sodium hypochlorite (bleach) to detergent solutions, or accelerated hydrogen peroxide solutions. Proper contact times should be used together with thorough handwashing.

Vaccines for FHV-1 and FCV have been available for several decades, but do not provide complete protection and disease continues to be widespread in the cat population. Infection of kittens before completion of the primary vaccine series occurs contributes to this problem. However, when infections are a problem in kittens in breeding catteries, vaccination of the queen before mating is preferable to vaccination during pregnancy, and may serve to prolong the duration of maternal antibody persistence.[50] Vaccination of kittens as early as 4 weeks of age could be considered in catteries that experience high rates of viral URTD. The primary series should consist of vaccines administered every 3 to 4 weeks of age until no earlier than 16 to 20 weeks of age.[51] None of the respiratory viral vaccines prevent infection, development of the carrier state, or reactivation of FHV-1 infection with stress, but they can reduce the severity of disease and the duration of shedding of FHV-1.[10,52,53] When all other control measures fail in breeding catteries, early weaning and isolation of kittens from 4 weeks of age could be considered.

REFERENCES

1. Helps CR, Lait P, Damhuis A, et al. Factors associated with upper respiratory tract disease caused by feline herpesvirus, feline calicivirus, Chlamydophila felis and Bordetella bronchiseptica in cats: experience from 218 European catteries. Vet Rec 2005;156:669–73.
2. Veir JK, Ruch-Gallie R, Spindel ME, et al. Prevalence of selected infectious organisms and comparison of two anatomic sampling sites in shelter cats with upper respiratory tract disease. J Feline Med Surg 2008;10:551–7.
3. Bech-Nielsen S, Fulton RW, Cox HU, et al. Feline respiratory tract disease in Louisiana. Am J Vet Res 1980;41:1293–8.
4. Ellis TM. Feline respiratory virus carriers in clinically healthy cats. Aust Vet J 1981;57:115–8.
5. Harbour DA, Howard PE, Gaskell RM. Isolation of feline calicivirus and feline herpesvirus from domestic cats 1980 to 1989. Vet Rec 1991;128:77–80.
6. Shewen PE, Povey RC, Wilson MR. A survey of the conjunctival flora of clinically normal cats and cats with conjunctivitis. Can Vet J 1980;21:231–3.
7. Wardley RC, Gaskell RM, Povey RC. Feline respiratory viruses: their prevalence in clinically healthy cats. J Small Anim Pract 1974;15:579–86.
8. Coutts AJ, Dawson S, Willoughby K, et al. Isolation of feline respiratory viruses from clinically healthy cats at UK cat shows. Vet Rec 1994;135:555–6.
9. Ruch-Gallie RA, Veir JK, Hawley JR, et al. Results of molecular diagnostic assays targeting feline herpesvirus-1 and feline calicivirus in adult cats administered modified live vaccines. J Feline Med Surg 2011;13:541–5.
10. Gaskell R, Dawson S, Radford A, et al. Feline herpesvirus. Vet Res 2007;38: 337–54.
11. Nasisse MP, Guy JS, Davidson MG, et al. Experimental ocular herpesvirus infection in the cat. Sites of virus replication, clinical features and effects of corticosteroid administration. Invest Ophthalmol Vis Sci 1989;30:1758–68.
12. Radford AD, Turner PC, Bennett M, et al. Quasispecies evolution of a hypervariable region of the feline calicivirus capsid gene in cell culture and in persistently infected cats. J Gen Virol 1998;79(Pt 1):1–10.
13. Doultree JC, Druce JD, Birch CJ, et al. Inactivation of feline calicivirus, a Norwalk virus surrogate. J Hosp Infect 1999;41:51–7.
14. Belgard S, Truyen U, Thibault JC, et al. Relevance of feline calicivirus, feline immunodeficiency virus, feline leukemia virus, feline herpesvirus and Bartonella henselae in cats with chronic gingivostomatitis. Berl Munch Tierarztl Wochenschr 2010;123:369–76.
15. Dowers KL, Hawley JR, Brewer MM, et al. Association of Bartonella species, feline calicivirus, and feline herpesvirus 1 infection with gingivostomatitis in cats. J Feline Med Surg 2010;12:314–21.
16. Hennet PR, Camy GA, McGahie DM, et al. Comparative efficacy of a recombinant feline interferon omega in refractory cases of calicivirus-positive cats with caudal stomatitis: a randomised, multi-centre, controlled, double-blind study in 39 cats. J Feline Med Surg 2011;13:577–87.

17. Hurley KE, Pesavento PA, Pedersen NC, et al. An outbreak of virulent systemic feline calicivirus disease. J Am Vet Med Assoc 2004;224:241–9.
18. Pedersen NC, Elliott JB, Glasgow A, et al. An isolated epizootic of hemorrhagic-like fever in cats caused by a novel and highly virulent strain of feline calicivirus. Vet Microbiol 2000;73:281–300.
19. Reynolds BS, Poulet H, Pingret JL, et al. A nosocomial outbreak of feline calicivirus associated virulent systemic disease in France. J Feline Med Surg 2009; 11:633–44.
20. Schulz BS, Hartmann K, Unterer S, et al. Two outbreaks of virulent systemic feline calicivirus infection in cats in Germany. Berl Munch Tierarztl Wochenschr 2011;124:186–93.
21. Radford AD, Gaskell RM. Dealing with a potential case of FCV-associated virulent systemic disease. Vet Rec 2011;168:585–6.
22. Coyne KP, Jones BR, Kipar A, et al. Lethal outbreak of disease associated with feline calicivirus infection in cats. Vet Rec 2006;158:544–50.
23. Pesavento PA, Stokol T, Liu H, et al. Distribution of the feline calicivirus receptor junctional adhesion molecule a in feline tissues. Vet Pathol 2011;48:361–8.
24. Poulet H. Virulent systemic calicivirus strains: what makes them so special? In: ISCAID-Merial ECVIM Pre-congress Symposium. Liverpool (United Kingdom), September 11, 2013. p. 33.
25. Sibitz C, Rudnay EC, Wabnegger L, et al. Detection of Chlamydophila pneumoniae in cats with conjunctivitis. Vet Ophthalmol 2011;14(Suppl 1):67–74.
26. Low HC, Powell CC, Veir JK, et al. Prevalence of feline herpesvirus 1, Chlamydophila felis, and Mycoplasma spp DNA in conjunctival cells collected from cats with and without conjunctivitis. Am J Vet Res 2007;68:643–8.
27. Binns SH, Speakman AJ, Dawson S, et al. The use of pulsed-field gel electrophoresis to examine the epidemiology of Bordetella bronchiseptica isolated from cats and other species. Epidemiol Infect 1998;120:201–8.
28. Dawson S, Jones D, McCracken CM, et al. Bordetella bronchiseptica infection in cats following contact with infected dogs. Vet Rec 2000;146:46–8.
29. Foley JE, Rand C, Bannasch MJ, et al. Molecular epidemiology of feline bordetellosis in two animal shelters in California, USA. Prev Vet Med 2002;54: 141–56.
30. Kirilenko NI. Survival of Bordetella pertussis in the air and on some objects. Zh Mikrobiol Epidemiol Immunobiol 1965;42:39–42 [in Russian].
31. Binns SH, Dawson S, Speakman AJ, et al. Prevalence and risk factors for feline Bordetella bronchiseptica infection. Vet Rec 1999;144:575–80.
32. Haesebrouck F, Devriese LA, van Rijssen B, et al. Incidence and significance of isolation of mycoplasma felis from conjunctival swabs of cats. Vet Microbiol 1991;26:95–101.
33. Holst BS, Hanas S, Berndtsson LT, et al. Infectious causes for feline upper respiratory tract disease: a case-control study. J Feline Med Surg 2010;12: 783–9.
34. Tillman PC, Dodson ND, Indiveri M. Group G streptococcal epizootic in a closed cat colony. J Clin Microbiol 1982;16:1057–60.
35. Britton AP, Davies JL. Rhinitis and meningitis in two shelter cats caused by Streptococcus equi subspecies zooepidemicus. J Comp Pathol 2010;143:70–4.
36. Blum S, Elad D, Zukin N, et al. Outbreak of Streptococcus equi subsp. zooepidemicus infections in cats. Vet Microbiol 2010;144:236–9.
37. Pesavento PA, Bannasch MJ, Bachmann R, et al. Fatal Streptococcus canis infections in intensively housed shelter cats. Vet Pathol 2007;44:218–21.

38. Goldschmidt P, Rostane H, Saint-Jean C, et al. Effects of topical anaesthetics and fluorescein on the real-time PCR used for the diagnosis of herpesviruses and *Acanthamoeba keratitis*. Br J Ophthalmol 2006;90:1354–6.
39. Maggs DJ. Antiviral therapy for feline herpesvirus infections. Vet Clin North Am Small Anim Pract 2010;40:1055–62.
40. Malik R, Lessels NS, Webb S, et al. Treatment of feline herpesvirus-1 associated disease in cats with famciclovir and related drugs. J Feline Med Surg 2009;11: 40–8.
41. Thomasy SM, Lim CC, Reilly CM, et al. Evaluation of orally administered famciclovir in cats experimentally infected with feline herpesvirus type-1. Am J Vet Res 2011;72:85–95.
42. Fontenelle JP, Powell CC, Veir JK, et al. Effect of topical ophthalmic application of cidofovir on experimentally induced primary ocular feline herpesvirus-1 infection in cats. Am J Vet Res 2008;69:289–93.
43. Maggs DJ. Ocular pharmacology and therapeutics. In: Maggs DJ, Miller PE, Ofri R, editors. Slatter's fundamentals of veterinary ophthalmology. 5th edition. St Louis (MO): Elsevier; 2013.
44. Sykes JE. Antiviral and immunomodulatory drugs. In: Sykes JE, editor. Canine and feline infectious diseases. 1st edition. St Louis (MO): Elsevier; 2014. p. 54–65.
45. Stiles J, Townsend WM, Rogers QR, et al. Effect of oral administration of L-lysine on conjunctivitis caused by feline herpesvirus in cats. Am J Vet Res 2002;63: 99–103.
46. Maggs DJ, Nasisse MP, Kass PH. Efficacy of oral supplementation with L-lysine in cats latently infected with feline herpesvirus. Am J Vet Res 2003;64:37–42.
47. Rees TM, Lubinski JL. Oral supplementation with L-lysine did not prevent upper respiratory infection in a shelter population of cats. J Feline Med Surg 2008;10: 510–3.
48. Bradley A, Kinyon J, Frana T, et al. Efficacy of intranasal administration of a modified live feline herpesvirus 1 and feline calicivirus vaccine against disease caused by *Bordetella bronchiseptica* after experimental challenge. J Vet Intern Med 2012;26:1121–5.
49. Tanaka A, Wagner DC, Kass PH, et al. Associations among weight loss, stress, and upper respiratory tract infection in shelter cats. J Am Vet Med Assoc 2012; 240:570–6.
50. Radford AD, Addie D, Belak S, et al. Feline calicivirus infection. ABCD guidelines on prevention and management. J Feline Med Surg 2009;11:556–64.
51. Scherk MA, Ford RB, Gaskell RM, et al. 2013 AAFP feline vaccination advisory panel report. J Feline Med Surg 2013;15:785–808.
52. Sykes JE, Browning GF, Anderson G, et al. Differential sensitivity of culture and the polymerase chain reaction for detection of feline herpesvirus 1 in vaccinated and unvaccinated cats. Arch Virol 1997;142:65–74.
53. Sussman MD, Maes RK, Kruger JM. Vaccination of cats for feline rhinotracheitis results in a quantitative reduction of virulent feline herpesvirus-1 latency load after challenge. Virology 1997;228:379–82.

Diagnosis and Management of Urinary Ectopia

Autumn P. Davidson, DVM, MS[a,b,*], Jodi L. Westropp, DVM, PhD[c]

KEYWORDS

- Ectopic ureter • Urinary incontinence • Diagnostics • Dogs • Ultrasonography
- Laser

KEY POINTS

- Ectopic ureters are the most common cause of urinary incontinence in young dogs but should be considered as a differential in any incontinent dog for which the history is not known.
- Ectopic ureters can be diagnosed with excretory urography, fluoroscopic urethrography or ureterography, abdominal ultrasonography, cystoscopy, helical computed tomography, or a combination of these diagnostic procedures. Other congenital abnormalities can also occur in dogs with ectopic ureters, including renal agenesis or dysplasia, hydronephrosis, and/or hydroureter and vestibulovaginal anomalies; therefore, the entire urinary system must be evaluated with ultrasonography if cystoscopy is the only other diagnostic tool used before surgery.
- Novel surgical techniques and adjunctive medical management have improved the prognosis for dogs with urinary ectopia.

 A video of laser revision of ectopic ureter accompanies this article at http://www.vetsmall.theclinics.com/

An *ectopic ureter* (EU) is defined as a ureteral opening that enters the urinary tract in any location other than the trigone of the bladder. In veterinary medicine, EUs are usually identified as entering distal to the trigone, and dogs usually present with varying degrees of urinary incontinence. EUs are the most common cause of urinary incontinence in young dogs but should be considered as a differential in any dog for which the history is not known. Although urinary incontinence is usually evident at weaning, clinical signs may not arise or be noted in some dogs until they have reached maturity. The severity of urinary incontinence is variable in dogs with EUs, and nocturia may be the only clinical sign. Breeds reported to be at risk include the golden retriever, Labrador retriever, Siberian Husky, Newfoundland, and English bulldog. The condition should be considered heritable (**Table 1**). EUs are uncommon in male dogs and, if

[a] Veterinary Medical Teaching Hospital Small Animal Clinic, Department of Medicine and Epidemiology, School of Veterinary Medicine, University of California, 1 Shields Avenue, Davis, CA 95616, USA; [b] Pet Care Veterinary Hospital, East Campus, 2425 Mendocino Avenue, Santa Rosa, CA 95403, USA; [c] Department of Medicine and Epidemiology, School of Veterinary Medicine, University of California, Davis, 2108 Tupper Hall, Davis, CA 95616, USA
* Corresponding author.
E-mail address: apdavidson@ucdavis.edu

Vet Clin Small Anim 44 (2014) 343–353
http://dx.doi.org/10.1016/j.cvsm.2013.11.007
0195-5616/14/$ – see front matter © 2014 Elsevier Inc. All rights reserved.

Table 1
Canine familial or heritable urinary tract disorders

Breed	Disorder	Trait
Alaskan malamute	Renal dysplasia	
Basenji	Fanconi syndrome	Familial
Bernese mountain dog	Membranoproliferative glomerulonephritis	Autosomal recessive
Beagle	Renal agenesis	Familial
	Membranoproliferative glomerulonephritis	Familial
Border terrier	Renal dysplasia	
	Fanconi syndrome	
Boxer	Renal dysplasia	Familial
Brie sheepdog	Renal dysplasia	
Brittany spaniel	Membranoproliferative glomerulonephritis	Autosomal recessive
Bull terrier	Glomerulopathy	Autosomal dominant
	Polycystic kidney	Autosomal dominant
Bulldog	Renal dysplasia	
Bullmastiff	Glomerulonephropathy	Autosomal recessive
	Renal dysplasia	
Cavalier King Charles spaniel	Renal agenesis	
	Xanthinuria	
	Renal dysplasia + agenesis	
Chinese Shar-Pei	Amyloidosis	
Chow-chow	Renal dysplasia	Familial
Cocker spaniel	Renal dysplasia: related?	
Dachshund	Xanthinuria	
Dalmatian	Glomerulopathy	Autosomal dominant
	Uric aciduria	Recessive
Doberman pinscher	Renal agenesis	Familial
	Glomerulopathy	Familial
Dutch Kooiker	Renal dysplasia	Familial
English bulldog	Renal and ureteral duplication	
	Uric aciduria	
	Ectopic ureter	
	Urethrorectal fistula	
English cocker spaniel	Glomerulopathy	Autosomal recessive
English foxhound	Amyloidosis	
Finnish harrier	Renal dysplasia	Familial
Fox terrier	Ectopic ureter	
German shepherd	Multifocal renal cystadenocarcinoma	Autosomal dominant
Golden retriever	Renal dysplasia	Familial
	Ectopic ureter	
Great Dane	Renal dysplasia	
Labrador retriever	Ectopic ureter	
Lhasa apso	Renal dysplasia	Familial

(continued on next page)

Table 1
(continued)

Breed	Disorder	Trait
Miniature poodle	Urethrorectal fistula, urethroperineal fistula, urethral duplication	
Miniature schnauzer	Renal dysplasia Fanconi syndrome	Familial
Newfoundland	Glomerulopathy Cystinuria Ectopic ureter	Familial Autosomal recessive
Norwegian elkhound	Fanconi syndrome	
Pekingese	Renal agenesis	
Pembroke Welsh corgi	Ectopic ureter Renal telangiectasia	
Poodle	Ectopic ureter	
Rhodesian ridgeback	Renal dysplasia	
Rottweiler	Glomerulopathy	Unknown
Samoyed	Renal dysplasia Glomerulopathy	X-linked
Scottish terrier	Cystinuria	Autosomal recessive
Shetland sheepdog	Renal agenesis Fanconi syndrome	Familial
Shih Tzu	Renal dysplasia	Familial
Siberian Husky	Ectopic ureter	
Skye terrier	Ectopic ureter	
Standard poodle	Renal dysplasia	Familial
West Highland white terrier	Ectopic ureter	
Soft-coated wheaten terrier	Renal dysplasia Membranoproliferative glomerulonephritis	Familial Familial

From Gordon J, Kutzler M. The urinary system. In: Peterson M, Kutzler M, editors. Small animal pediatrics: the first 12 months of age. Philadelphia: Elsevier; 2011. p. 395; with permission.

present, these animals often will not have clinical signs.[1] This fact could be because of the increased length of the urethra in male dogs. EUs are extremely rare in cats.

EUs can be intramural or extramural, with the former being far more common in dogs. More than 95% of EUs are reported to be intramural. Intramural EUs are defined as ureters that enter the bladder in a normal location; however, they tunnel in the submucosa and extend distal to the trigone, opening in various locations along the genitourinary tract.[2] Intramural EUs are well described in human beings and thought to occur because of the failure of migration or absorption of the ureteral bud and common excretory duct; therefore, the opening of the ureter will be positioned along the path of the ureteral migration. Data evaluating EUs cystoscopically in dogs support this theory in canines.[3] EUs in dogs and cats have been reported to result from failed migration of the metanephros from the sacral region of the embryo during the final stage of development of the urinary system.[4] Extramural EUs bypass the trigone altogether and enter somewhere in the distal genitourinary tract. Extramural EUs result from failure of the mesonephric duct to contact the urogenital sinus.

EUs can be diagnosed with excretory urography, fluoroscopic urethrography or ureterography, abdominal ultrasonography, cystoscopy, helical computed tomography (CT), or a combination of these diagnostic procedures. Helical CT and cystoscopy are reported to be the most sensitive diagnostics for identifying EUs.[3,5] In older studies, unilateral EUs were documented more often; however, when cystoscopy was used to define the ectopics, bilateral ureters appeared more often. This finding is likely because of the more aggressive definition of an EU and closer visual inspection of the trigone area.

Cystoscopy is also beneficial because it allows one to visualize the vestibule and genitourinary mucosa for other abnormalities, such as persistent paramesonephric remnants, vestibulovaginal septate bands, dual vagina, or even vestibulovaginal ectopics that occur rarely (**Figs. 1** and **2**). Cystoscopy also permits identification of urachal diverticuli, which can occur with EUs (**Fig. 3**).

Other congenital abnormalities can also occur in dogs with EUs, including renal agenesis or dysplasia, hydronephrosis, and/or hydroureter; therefore, the entire urinary system must be evaluated with ultrasonography if cystoscopy is the only other diagnostic used before surgery. Dilation of the ureter improves the sensitivity of the ultrasound study; however, the diagnosis can be elusive. Visualization of a nonvascular fluid-filled structure with a hyperechoic wall passing dorsal to the urinary bladder, or the obvious insertion of the structure into the proximal urethra, suggest the diagnosis (**Fig. 4**). Visualization of only the ureteral jets in the bladder suggests normalcy; however, some EUs insert initially into the bladder and additionally tunnel distally to terminate in an abnormal site (**Fig. 5**). The normal ureterovesicular junction (at the ureteral papilla) appears as a slight thickening of the urinary bladder mucosa, if visible at all (**Fig. 6**). More commonly, only the ureteral jet is seen as urine enters the bladder. Visualization of distinct ureteral walls, which contain smooth muscle and display pulsatile motion, suggests ureteral abnormality, such as ectopia. This irregularity can uncommonly be observed with intensive diuresis or severe urinary outflow obstruction distal to the ureter in otherwise normal dogs (**Fig. 7**). Observation of the EU usually occurs near the urinary bladder. Visualization of the bladder neck and proximal urethra may be obscured by the pubic bone, making identification of this

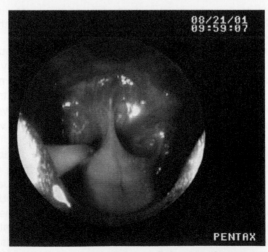

Fig. 1. Vaginoscopic appearance of a septate vestibular band positioned just cranial to the urethral papilla.

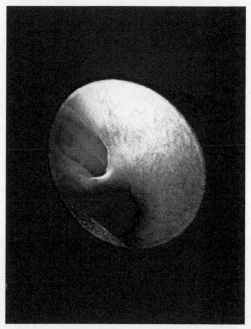

Fig. 2. Cystoscopic appearance of the entrance of an EU into the cranial vestibule. The vestibulovaginal junction is seen to the right.

termination difficult. Hydroureter and hydronephrosis can eventually result from an uncorrected EU caused by flow impedance at the abnormal site of insertion (**Fig. 8**). Urinary tract infection (UTI) is commonly associated with ectopia, because of accompanying urethral sphincter mechanism anomalies, and if not detected and treated can progress to pyelonephritis and ureteritis. Infection and its associated inflammation in

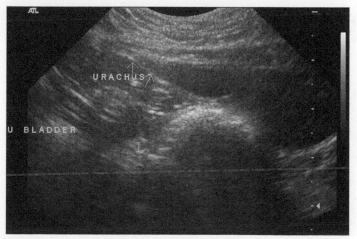

Fig. 3. Sagittal ultrasound image of a urachal diverticulum (*arrows*) at the urinary bladder apex. (*Courtesy of* Dr TW Baker, Davis, CA.)

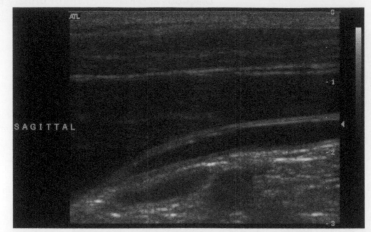

Fig. 4. Sagittal ultrasound image of bilateral, dilated EUs (*arrow head*) coursing dorsal to the bladder trigone. (*Courtesy of* Dr TW Baker, Davis, CA.)

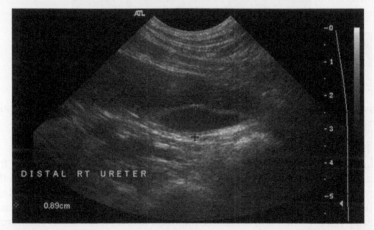

Fig. 5. Transverse ultrasound image of an intramural right dilated EU (*cursors*). (*Courtesy of* Dr TW Baker, Davis, CA.)

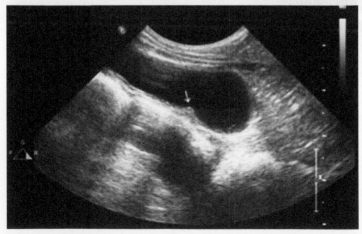

Fig. 6. Sagittal ultrasound image of a normal ureterovesicular junction (*arrow*). (*Courtesy of* Dr Eric Johnson, Davis, CA.)

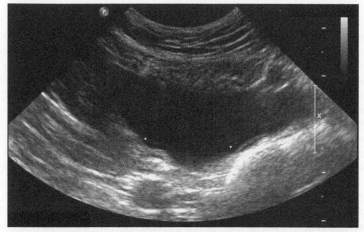

Fig. 7. Transverse ultrasound image of normal ureterovesicular junctions exhibiting fluid distension secondary to intensive diuresis (*dots*). (*Courtesy of* Dr Eric Johnson, Davis, CA.)

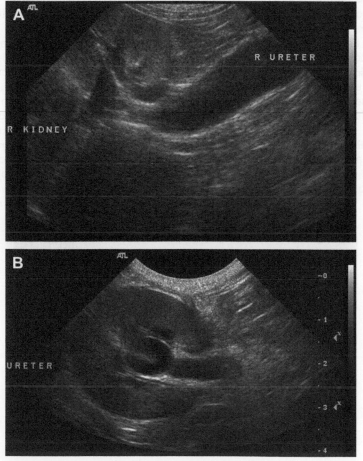

Fig. 8. Transverse ultrasonographic image of (*A*) hydroureter and (*B*) hydronephrosis resulting from an uncorrected right EU. (*Courtesy of* Dr TW Baker, Davis, CA.)

the tract can further alter the ultrasonographic appearance of the kidneys, bladder, ureters, and urethra, and underscores the importance of including ultrasonography in the preoperative diagnostics. A ureterocele is a congenital dilation of the ureter near the bladder, appearing as a cystic structure within the bladder lumen or wall. The ureterocele occurs most commonly in association with an EU. It can be diagnosed through scanning the urinary bladder wall in the transverse plane and watching for strong peristalsis of the ureterocele (**Fig. 9**).

Because UTIs occur frequently in dogs with EUs, urine cultures should always be performed in dogs with suspected EUs. Early diagnosis of EU and intervention is desirable in pediatric dogs; progression to hydroureter, hydronephrosis, bacterial cystitis, and pyelonephritis occurs with high frequency if untreated (**Fig. 10**). Irreversible renal damage can occur. Preoperative evaluation should include a complete blood cell count, biochemical profile, and urinalysis with culture and sensitivity, obtained ideally via percutaneous ultrasound-guided cystocentesis. A negative urine culture is desirable preoperatively. Perivulvar dermatitis associated with incontinence should be treated if present (**Fig. 11**). Urodynamics, often available only at academic or specialty practices, can provide information about urethral sphincter tone and predict to some extent the prognosis for continence after revision.

Traditionally, treatment for dogs with ureteral ectopia is surgical correction, and postoperative success rates vary between 50% and 75%.[6] Dogs weighing less than 20 kg have been reported to have a better outcome postoperatively.[6] The poor success rate could be from a variety of causes, including incorrectly identifying the terminal portion of the EU, the presence of multiple ureteral openings, concurrent urethral sphincter mechanism incompetence, or a combination of these. Surgical techniques include ureteroneocystostomy (transection of the EU distally with anastomosis of the proximal portion to the urinary bladder, usually reserved for extramural ectopia), neoureterostomy with ligation of the distal ectopic segment, neoureterostomy with resection of the distal ectopic segment and revision of the trigone and urethra, and nephrectomy (usually reserved for intractable hydronephrosis or pyelonephritis or in cases with severe financial constraints). Postoperative complications include persistent incontinence, hydronephrosis, and the risks associated with open

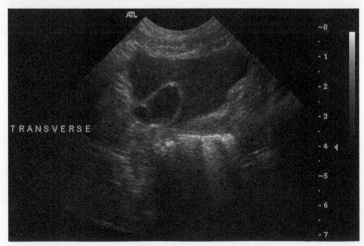

Fig. 9. Transverse ultrasound image of a unilateral ureterocele (larger structure) and EU. (*Courtesy of* Dr TW Baker, Davis, CA.)

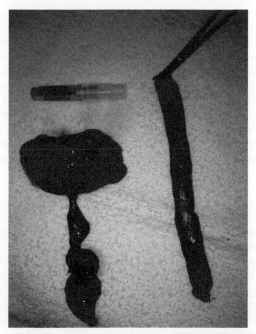

Fig. 10. Gross specimens following nephrectomy in a 9-month old Labrador retriever with chronic pyelonephritis resulting from an uncorrected right ectopic ureter. The kidney (below needle) had irreversible damage and served as a nidus of infection. A section of the distal EU is seen to the right.

abdominal surgery. Persistent incontinence is likely caused by the trough effect of the remaining intraurethral ureteral remnant left behind because of surgical inaccessibility.[7]

Minimally invasive therapies have also been used in dogs with EUs, such as cystoscopic-guided laser ablation for the EU (**Fig. 12** and Video 1). This technique is used to treat intramural EUs in either male or female dogs.[8,9] Preliminary reports suggest that urinary continence after this procedure is comparable or better than after

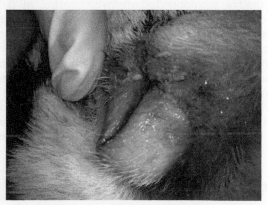

Fig. 11. Perivulvar moist dermatitis and pyoderma associated with urine scalding resulting from chronic urinary incontinence secondary to EU.

surgery, but too few cases have been occurred to fully evaluate long-term outcome.[8,9] For this procedure, the dog is anesthetized and positioned in either right lateral, sternal, or dorsal recumbency, depending on the clinician's preference. Cystoscopy and vaginoscopy are performed using passive saline (0.9% sodium chloride) insufflation through a rigid cystourethroscope (1.9–4.0 mm). Many clinicians also prefer to perform this procedure using fluoroscopy, if available, and therefore additional ureteral studies can be obtained during the procedure, if necessary, to confirm that the ureter is intramural. Once an intramural EU has been identified, a 4-French open-ended ureteral catheter is inserted over a 0.35 mm flexible weasel wire to protect the lateral ureteral wall. Various laser fibers can be used to cut the ectopic tunnel, depending on what is available to the clinician. Although a diode laser provides a cleaner cut, the authors use the holmium:yttrium, aluminum, and garnet laser, which also works very well for this procedure, however the cuts are not as continuous and the higher settings are needed as the tissue becomes thicker. Alternatively, transection can be accomplished using a radiofrequency surgical device. The ectopic tunnel is cut as far back to the trigone as possible, but care must be taken to not continue the incision as the ureter becomes extramural in nature. Vestibulovaginal septate bands, if present, should be transacted, because they can contribute to incontinence and discomfort by displacing the urethral papilla dorsally (see **Fig. 8**).

In a small case series of 12 female dogs, continence was achieved in 47% of dogs without additional medical management (Westropp, DVM, PhD, personal communication). When pharmacologic intervention (eg, phenylpropanolamine or estrogen compounds) were added, continence increased to 77% of dogs. All owners were satisfied with the procedure, and 87% were extremely satisfied. Advantages for this minimally invasive procedure include the possibility of a quicker recovery time, and lack of problems associated with a midline incision (eg, need for Elizabethan collar, restricted activity). Some dogs seem to experience some vulvovaginal irritation, which can be managed with oral nonsteroidal anti-inflammatory drugs or narcotics. The option of ovariectomy or ovariohysterectomy performed at the same time as EU revision is lost unless performed laparoscopically when the cystoscopic approach is used. Removal of affected individuals from breeding programs should always be discussed with the owners.

Postoperative persistent incontinence can be managed in many cases pharmacologically with the α-adrenergic stimulant phenylpropanolamine (1.0–1.5 mg/kg orally every 8–12 hours), or estrogen compounds that increase sensitivity of α-adrenergic receptors in the urethra (compounded diethylstilboestrol at 0.02 mg/kg orally, tapered to 1 to 3 times weekly or estriol at 2 mg orally given daily, then tapered). Time-released phenylpropanolamine is more effective than the short-acting formulation in refractory cases of incontinence. Combination therapy with phenylpropanolamine and an estrogen compound can be superior if either fails as a single agent. Gonadotropin-releasing hormone (GnRH) analogues were recently shown to improve continence in ovariectomized female dogs, most likely through interaction with GnRH, follicle-stimulating hormone, and luteinizing hormone receptors in the lower genitourinary tract.[10] A postoperative urine culture should always be determined before assuming that persistent incontinence is caused by residual anatomic abnormalities.

SUPPLEMENTARY DATA

Supplementary data related to this article can be found online at http://dx.doi.org/10.1016/j.cvsm.2013.11.007.

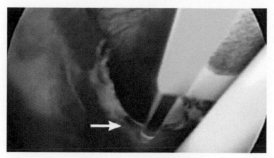

Fig. 12. Laser ablation of the medial wall of the intramural portion of an ectopic ureter (*arrow*).

REFERENCES

1. Holt P, Moore A. Canine ureteral ectopia: an analysis of 175 cases and comparison of surgical treatments. Vet Rec 1995;136(14):345–9.
2. Lautzenhiser S, Bjorling D. Urinary incontinence in a dog with an ectopic ureterocele. J Am Anim Hosp Assoc 2002;38(1):29–32.
3. Cannizzo K, McLoughlin M, Mattoon J, et al. Evaluation of transurethral cystoscopy and excretory urography for diagnosis of ectopic ureters in female dogs: 25 cases (1992-2000). J Am Vet Med Assoc 2003;223(4):475–81.
4. Gordon J, Kutzler M. The urinary system. In: Peterson M, Kutzler M, editors. Small animal pediatrics: the first 12 months of age. St Louis, MO: Elsevier; 2011. p. 391–404.
5. Samii V, McLoughlin M, Mattoon J, et al. Digital fluoroscopic excretory urography, digital fluoroscopic urethrography, helical computed tomography, and cystoscopy in 24 dogs with suspected ureteral ectopia. J Vet Intern Med 2004;18(3): 271–81.
6. Smith C, Stowater J, Kneller S. Ectopic ureter in the dog-a review of cases. J Am Anim Hosp Assoc 1981;17:245–8.
7. Stone E, Mason L. Surgery of ectopic ureters: types, method of correction, and postoperative results. J Am Anim Hosp Assoc 1990;26:81–8.
8. Berent AC, Mayhew PD, Porat-Mosenco Y. Use of cystoscopic-guided laser ablation for treatment of intramural ureteral ectopia in male dogs: four cases (2006-2007). J Am Vet Med Assoc 2008;232(7):1026–34. http://dx.doi.org/10. 2460/javma.232.7.1026.
9. Berent A, Weisse C, Mayhew P, et al. Evaluation of cystoscopic-guided laser ablation of intramural ectopic ureters in female dogs. J Am Vet Med Assoc 2012;240(6):716–25.
10. Reichler IM, Jochle W, Piché CA, et al. Effect of a long acting GnRH analogue or placebo on plasma LH/FSH, urethral pressure profiles and clinical signs of urinary incontinence due to sphincter mechanism incompetence in bitches. Theriogenology 2006;66(5):1227–36.

Holistic Pediatric Veterinary Medicine

Lisa Pesch, DVM With Thesis

KEYWORDS

- Holistic • Pediatric • Veterinary medicine • Treatment

KEY POINTS

- An increasing number of clients are seeking holistic care for their pets.
- Holistic veterinary medicine treats the whole patient including all physical and behavioral clinical signs.
- Herbal and nutritional supplements can help support tissue healing and proper organ functioning, thereby reducing the tendency toward disease progression over time.
- Many herbal and nutraceutical companies provide support for veterinarians, assisting with proper formula selection, dosing, drug interactions, and contraindications.

HOLISTIC PERSPECTIVE

Holistic medicine is a way of practicing not a modality. *Holistic* is defined as "characterized by comprehension of the parts of something as intimately interconnected and explicable only by reference to the whole."[1] In medicine, the term is also used to describe the treatment of the whole patient, including physical, mental, and social symptoms of a disease. A veterinarian can practice as holistically as possible regardless of the techniques they use. However, some modalities lend themselves much more readily to a holistic approach than others. Therefore, practitioners interested in using a holistic approach will benefit greatly from learning these modalities.

Individual Nature of Health and Disease

As veterinarians, we see some patients only for routine examinations and vaccinations, whereas others present repeatedly for ailments. These patients' ailments often relapse when treatments are discontinued. Sometimes a patient exhibits a specific pattern of disease that moves from one location to another. For example, one might see a puppy for vaginitis, later otitis externa, and then subsequently for enteritis. A sudden onset of inflammation, odor, pain, and discharge might be present in this

Animal Healing Arts, PO Box 14625, Santa Rosa, CA 95402, USA; Pet Care Veterinary Hospital, East Campus, Holistic Medicine, 2425 Mendocino Avenue, Santa Rosa, CA 95403, USA; Veterinary Technology Program, Agriculture & Natural Resources, Santa Rosa Junior College, 1501 Mendocino Avenue, Santa Rosa, CA 95401, USA
E-mail address: info@lisapeschdvm.com

Vet Clin Small Anim 44 (2014) 355–366
http://dx.doi.org/10.1016/j.cvsm.2013.11.003
vetsmall.theclinics.com

patient each time, whereas another individual might experience slow smoldering signs and lethargy whenever sick.

Progression of Disease

Most veterinarians are well educated in proper diagnostic methods and judicious use of medications. A cat presenting with signs of cystitis only receives antibiotics if warranted by a urinalysis. Using thorough diagnostic protocols to select appropriate medicines often leaves simpler effective treatment lacking for relatively common maladies. Relapses of a condition after discontinuing medication can be concerning. Diarrhea might respond quickly to a bland diet and kaolin and then relapse needing more extended treatment. With time, the returning condition may require strong medicines (with significant potential side effects) to achieve what 3 days of a bland diet had initially achieved. Even with proper treatment, sign severity often progresses from very mild to severe over time. We can often predict the pattern of progression without effectively averting it. The only choice seems to sequentially apply increased suppression to the signs. The temptation arises to apply the big guns to the first outbreak of mild imbalance. This practice often extends the time until the signs return. However, when they do recur, their severity may increase more rapidly.

Treating Whole Patients

Through studying alternative therapies, one can become proficient in simpler yet effective forms of treatment that nourish patients (and their organs) and reverse this tendency to worsening. These techniques address all aspects of a patient's illnesses at the same time. A cat that often vomits, has a greasy coat with pruritus, is anxious with a tendency to become irritable, and presents for sterile cystitis no longer has 3 to 4 separate conditions. Improvement of each sign that is being treated is assessed but not as if separate from the others or the overall wellbeing of the patient. Signs are clues to the big picture of patient's basic imbalance or weakness. Their expression is related to one another as is their treatment. The author presents a very brief overview of modalities she uses as well as some basic treatments that may be useful for beginning holistic practitioners and conventional practitioners interested in integrating a new holistic approach into their practice.

DESCRIPTION OF COMMON COMPLEMENTARY AND ALTERNATIVE VETERINARY MEDICINE MODALITIES
Traditional Chinese (Veterinary) Medicine

Diagnosis and treatment using Traditional Chinese Medicine (TCM) emphasizes the functional aspects of health and disease. Disorders are grouped based on which organs are affected as well as the nature of the affection. Some practitioners are confused by the English translation of descriptive terms used in categorization. Some disregard the modality as valid because of its attempt to acknowledge conundrums and alternating states, whereas others find this one of its biggest strengths. Recognizing that terminology is merely an attempt to describe what is routinely seen clinically is exceedingly helpful. Reading a TCM colleague's diagnosis of toxic heat may sound exceedingly foreign; but when viewed as a description of the functional disturbances occurring within the body, this can be more readily understood. This label would be appropriate in conditions such as food poisoning or upper respiratory infections. It is an acknowledgment that the condition is creating increased heat in the body (as we know inflammation/infection does). It is also recognizing that the level of toxins in the body is high. We recognize that inflammation creates toxins; we can see toxic neutrophils on a complete blood count, and we can identify toxins caused or released by pathogenic organisms.

Traditional Chinese (veterinary) medicine terminology
Some examples of terms correlated with conventional medical concepts are listed next. These terms have been simplified and are not intended to provide a comprehensive understanding of the concepts they describe.

Qi: active metabolic expression and movement (potential and consumed energy)
Yin: substance, fluid, cold, inactivity, anabolism
Yang: insubstantial functional energy, dry, heat, activity, catabolism; qi that is heated up
Damp: fluid accumulation (ie, cellulitis, ascites, edema)
Wind: signs sudden and changeable, involve movement, or move around the body (ie, seizures, pruritus, wandering limb pain), acute infections
Phlegm: mucus, congealed accumulations, tumors
(Blood or qi) stagnation: a blockage of normal homeostasis or metabolism resulting in uneven distribution of microcirculation causing areas of deficiency and/or pooling
Deficiency: weakness, insufficiency
Excess: overactivity

Treatment using the traditional Chinese (veterinary) medicine model
Herbs and acupuncture point stimulation are studied in relation to their effects using functional categorization. *Bupleurum* has antiinflammatory, antipyretic, and edema-protective effects on the liver.[2] In TCM, it is described as a cooling herb for the liver that relieves liver stagnation.[3] Proper selection of herbal formulas depends on the practitioner's ability to properly diagnose (categorize) the condition. Treatment of dermatitis characterized by pruritus and dandruff in chilly, anxious, thirsty patients will require a different formula than dermatitis involving moist eruptions and odor in irritable/aggressive thirstless patients who easily overheat.

Homeopathy

Law of similars
Samuel Hahnemann discovered homeopathy in the late 1800s. Hahnemann was a medical physician with expertise in chemistry. He wrote a standard chemistry text and translated many medical texts. While translating a text, he noted that the effectiveness of cinchona in the treatment of malaria was attributed to its bitter and astringent qualities. He questioned this assessment recognizing that other bitter and astringent substances had no effect on malaria. Curious as to its action, he took cinchona and developed symptoms similar to that of malaria, which subsided when the herb was discontinued. This experience led him to hypothesize that it was instead the fact that the herb stimulated a similar reaction as the disease that catalyzed improvement in patients with malaria.[4-6] He performed extensive clinical trials administering substances to healthy individuals and recording the symptoms that were repeatedly induced. He used this information along with the known effects of the substances (ie, primary effects and side effects of medications) to select medicines. By administering medicine known to cause a particular set of symptoms to patients suffering from similar ailments, he found this form of treatment to be effective.

Medicinal (primary) action induces curative (counter) action
This effect correlates with our knowledge of homeostatic mechanisms. The homeopathic medicine, being similar to (mimicking) the disease, will increase the

homeostatic imbalance. This imbalance stimulates a response within the body to maintain balance. With homeopathic prescribing, substances with a short duration of action are used. Once the medicine is no longer active in the body, the heightened counteraction can more effectively restore health.

Medicine selection

Homeopathic prescribing is determined solely by signs. Signs are matched as specifically as possible to the signs known to be treated by the medicine. The more detailed the correlation, the more likely the remedy will initiate the physiologic reactions needed to restore homeostasis. A conventional diagnosis is included, but treatment often varies as does the sign expression of individual patients with a given diagnosis. For example, a kitten with a herpes virus infection causing thick yellow oculonasal discharge and sneezing requires a different prescription than one with increased thirst, corneal ulceration, and clear oculonasal discharge that irritates the tissues it contacts. Because proper treatment selection depends on sign evaluation, homeopathy is not compatible with treatments that strongly suppress or alter patients' signs.

Homeopathy definitions

Many clients frequently misuse the term *homeopathy*. They will often use it to describe any natural or alternative medicine (ie, herbal, nutraceuticals). Many laypersons as well as practitioners will use the term *homeopathy* to describe any use of substances that have been prepared homeopathically. Homeopathic preparation of substances involves extended vigorous agitation and succussion of the substance, which causes repeated molecular collisions, changing their electromagnetic dynamics. When Hahnemann coined the termed *homeopathy*, he meant it to describe the method of treatment using medicines that induced signs similar to the disease as described previously. Late in his career, Hahnemann developed the homeopathic preparation of substances and then focused his clinical trials on their use; his earlier clinical trials using homeopathy involved substances common to medical practice of the time, which would have been prepared conventionally. Hahnemann used the term *allopathy* to describe the use of medicines whose effects do not match patients' symptoms. Because of the confusion created by practitioners describing widely varying techniques as *homeopathy*, many people now use the term *classical homeopathy* to denote the original definition given to homeopathy.

Chiropractic Therapy

Chiropractic is the use of specific manipulations to the spine and extremities to restore range of motion. Range-of-motion palpation of all joints is performed to determine the location of hypomobile and/or hypermobile joints. There are a wide variety of chiropractic techniques available to restore normal range of motion in patients. A modified Gonstead technique is likely the most commonly used in animals. This technique involves the application of a low-impact, high-velocity thrust at a specific contact point in a specific line of drive to gently increase the range of motion to hypomobile areas. In spinal areas, the restoration of range of motion has secondary effects, including improved nerve conduction, improved nutrient delivery to intervertebral disks, and increased toxin clearance from tissues.

Manual Therapy

Other hands-on methods to restore normal musculoskeletal and spinal nerve functioning include the application of digital pressure to spinal lever points, using digital pressure to initiate reflex relaxation of tightened muscles, isometric stretches to restore normal muscle tone, acupressure, and massage. The goals of these techniques are generally to remove abnormal tension patterns, alleviate abnormal nerve conduction, improve tissue circulation, alleviate pain, and restore freedom of movement. In addition to the physical responses seen with these treatments, significant improvement in emotional and behavioral disorders can be seen. How grumpy are you with a stiff and painful neck?

TREATMENT OF DISEASES IN PEDIATRIC PATIENTS
Gastroenteritis

In puppies and kittens, diarrhea and vomiting are most commonly associated with viral infections, bacterial infections, endoparasites, dietary sensitivities, and dietary indiscretion.[7,8] Signs vary from mild to life threatening. The holistic approach treats the signs of gastroenteritis while at the same time attempting to eliminate the root cause. In the case of infectious and parasitic gastroenteritis, treatment addresses the imbalance leading to susceptibility. In the case of dietary sensitivity, it addresses the abnormal immune function; in indiscretions, it addresses the abnormal hunger that led to the unhealthy consumption. It is important to evaluate the location most affected in a given individual in order to identify organs that exhibit deficiencies. For example, in a litter of puppies showing a positive fecal evaluation for ascarids, one individual may show poor weight gain, another severe diarrhea, another vomiting, another vomiting and diarrhea, and another may be normal. From a holistic perspective, each of these individuals requires a different treatment plan.

Infection-associated gastroenteritis
In puppies and kittens life threatening disease is commonly associated with viral infections. Parvovirus type 1 is considered pathogenic in puppies under 6 weeks old.[9,10] Parvovirus type 2 and distemper virus are more commonly seen in puppies 6 weeks and older. In kittens common viruses associated with vomiting and diarrhea are feline panleukopenia, feline infectious peritonitis, feline leukemia virus, and feline immunodeficiency virus.[7,8] As morbidity for all viral diseases is less than 100%, individuals must be susceptible to an organism to develop signs. Healthy individuals with proper nourishment and husbandry born to a healthy immune dam or queen have lower susceptibility to these viruses. Thorough history taking regarding the previous health of the patient, health of the patient's mother, husbandry, health of littermates, and nursing/dietary intake will help to identify individuals at higher risk. Appropriately timed vaccination of healthy individuals will help to reduce the risk to severe life-threatening signs. It stands to reason that patients with susceptibility to a given virus would have increased susceptibility to the virus introduced in an altered form (vaccine). In these patients, acute manifestation of pathogenic infection may be avoided via vaccination; however, care should be taken to monitor for and treat any subacute signs correlated with vaccination, such as otitis, ocular discharge, skin eruptions, vomiting, or diarrhea.

Bacterial infections, similar to viral infections, result in susceptible hosts. Most bacteria associated with vomiting and diarrhea in puppies and kittens can be found in normal carriers. Puppies and kittens are more likely to exhibit severe signs in correlation with positive pathogenic fecal bacterial cultures or a polymerase chain reaction than adults.

Endoparasite-associated gastroenteritis
Endoparasites are associated with diarrhea, lack of weight gain, vomiting, bloating, and, in some cases, anemia (ie, hookworms and whipworms).[7,8,11] As with most causes of gastroenteritis, signs may vary from normal carriers to life-threatening illness.

Helminth Infestations

Ascarids are ubiquitous in the environment, and can be transmitted transplacentally and transmammary.[7,8,11] Puppies and kittens are routinely treated prophylactically for helminth infestations postnatally. Studies of stray dog populations show a decrease in prevalence of ascarid infections with increased age.[11–15] Adult individuals also tended to have lighter worm loads indicating natural immunity.[14,15] Individuals with difficult-to-clear or recurrent infestations should be evaluated for chronic disease.

Protozoal Infections

Giardia is normally encountered in the environment, and its presence does not indicate that it is the cause of signs.[7,11,16] Heavy overgrowths of this organism can contribute to signs and tissue damage.

Coccidial infections are generally self-limiting, and overgrowth of these organisms is generally secondary in nature.

Treatment of Gastroenteritis

Viral-, bacterial-, and endoparasite-associated diarrhea is most effectively treated by reducing the patients' susceptibility, protecting tissues from injury, and supporting the healing of damaged tissues. Holistically speaking, the disease occurs before infection or infestation. The question arises as to whether the initial damage to tissues is a result of pathogenic organism reproduction or if the reproduction of pathogenic organisms is made possible by damaged tissue. Regardless, the methods of treatment that restore health to damaged tissue will reduce organism reproduction and reverse impairments. Therefore, the practitioner may find it more useful to view these conditions as overgrowth rather than infections or infestations. The primary focus of treatment is restoring an environment within the patient that is no longer supportive for pathogenic organisms.

The treatment of underlying health issues, correcting husbandry deficiencies, and reducing stress before exposure will help reduce susceptibility to infections and parasitism. For patients presenting with evidence of existing infection or parasitism, proper treatment to reduce susceptibility will result in more rapid and effective resolution of infection with fewer residual signs. Although methods to reduce the number of pathogenic organisms or parasites are used as needed, restoration of normal immune system and gastrointestinal (GI) tract function is often all that is required to clear signs and associated organisms. Methods of treatment with the mildest side effects are chosen. In addition, treatments that strongly suppress signs without resulting in improved tissue health are discouraged. By using these methods, the patients' susceptibility remains unchanged or may, in fact, worsen. As a result, relapse on discontinuation of such methods or repeated infections are common.

Homeopathics, Herbals and Nutritional Supplements

Homeopathy has an advantage in patients with inappetence and medication avoidance because dosing is generally less frequent and homeopathic remedies are relatively tasteless. They are available in forms that allow for the easy administration and absorption without causing upset in patients who can have nothing by mouth. The remedy that best fits the signs in the patients is used.

Slippery elm is demulcent, emollient, and soothing to the alimentary canal.[2,17] Unfortunately, slippery elm populations are dwindling because of overharvesting for herbal use.[18] Ethical wild crafters recommend first gauging the amount needed and then stripping the bark from one-fourth or less of the branches.[18]

Marshmallow root is often used as an eco-friendly alternative to slippery elm. It contains bioadhesive and mucilaginous polysaccharides that create a mucinlike coating on irritated tissues.[19] It has also been shown to have antibacterial activity against pathogenic bacteria.[20,21] It has anticomplementary activity.[2] This fact may be beneficial in allergic, sensitivity, and noninfectious inflammatory states but raises concerns about its use during the active phase of viral infections. It has immune-stimulating effects and stimulates phagocytosis,[2] which may help to offset the effects of the anticomplementary activity. It has a hypoglycemic effect.[2]

Pill curing (Kang ning wan) treats nausea, vomiting, and diarrhea.[22–24] It is especially useful in dietary indiscretions and other acute forms of gastroenteritis. Pill curing has also been shown to have an effect against protozoal infections. The classic formula is not intended for long-term use. Modifications of this formula appropriate for chronic administration are available. These formulations can also be useful in reducing the GI effects of other herbs or medications.

Colostrum has been shown to promote proliferation and migration of gastric and small intestinal cells.[25,26] It has been shown to reduce gastric injury and villus shortening caused by nonsteroidal antiinflammatory drug administration.[25] It shows immune modulating and antibacterial effects. It neutralizes lipopolysaccharide endotoxins.[27]

Adjunctive therapy

A highly digestible diet relieves stress on the GI tract by reducing the demand for digestive enzymes. It reduces the amount of undigested food particles entering the colon. This reduction helps to minimize colonic irritability.

Acupuncture has antiemetic, antinausea, and appetite-stimulating effects. It is an effective pain reliever and promotes normal immune functioning.

Infection-Associated Respiratory Disease

The most common respiratory diseases in puppies are canine infectious respiratory disease (CIRD) also known as *kennel cough complex*. The organisms associated with CIRD in puppies are *Bordetella bronchiseptica* bacteria, parainfluenza virus, mycoplasma, adenovirus, distemper virus, influenza virus, and respiratory corona virus.[28,29] In kittens, upper respiratory infections are commonly associated with herpes virus 1 and calicivirus.[29] Secondary bacterial overgrowth may result from these infections. Puppies and kittens generally have a higher risk of infection compared with adults. Signs vary from mild to life threatening.

CIRD

The common signs of CIRD in puppies are a harsh hacking to honking cough often accompanied by tracheal sensitivity and gagging or retching of expectoration. Other signs that may be present are oculonasal discharge and sneezing with or without fever. Most patients will remain healthy in appearance with a normal appetite and activity levels. In some patients, the signs may progress to a secondary bronchopneumonia. These patients are more likely to exhibit lethargy and abnormal respiratory parameters. Diagnosis is generally based on clinical signs and history of exposure to other dogs. Transmission is by aerosol and fomites. Dogs housed in close quarters in large numbers (ie, kennels and shelters) are at higher risk.

Treatment of CIRD

The treatments for CIRD are focused at restoring immune function, reducing airway inflammation, alleviating cough, and supporting tissue healing.

Herbal supplements

Gan mao ling: This herbal formula reduces inflammation of the pharynx and upper trachea. It also promotes clearance of mucous accumulation.[17,21–23]

Ehr chen wan: This herbal formula dispels mucus, especially from the lower respiratory tract.[17,21–23] The initial response may be accompanied by symptoms associated with increased mobilization of thinner expectoration. If this creates significant patient discomfort, the dosage should be reduced to the desired effect.

Frittilary and loquat syrup: It reduces the cough with associated tracheal irritation and clears expectoration.[17,21]

Feline upper respiratory infections

Upper respiratory infections are common in kittens. Susceptibility to these organisms as well as the severity of signs in the individual is affected by age, nutrition status, husbandry, and coexisting disease. The common signs are sneezing and nasal discharge. Ocular lesions including conjunctivitis and corneal ulcers are associated with herpes virus infections. Calicivirus is associated with oral ulceration. Feline immunodeficiency virus and feline leukemia virus cause immunosuppression and may contribute to the severity or longevity of signs. In addition, alterations in immune function, mucus viscosity, mucociliary clearance, and tissue integrity associated with any of the aforementioned viruses can lead to secondary bacterial overgrowth.

Treatments for Feline Upper Respiratory Disease

Treatments are focused at restoring immune function, normalizing mucus viscosity and clearance, maintaining appetite, supporting tissue healing, and reducing scar-tissue formation.

Homeopathics, herbals and nutritional supplements

Homeopathy has an advantage in patients with oral pain or inappetence because dosing is generally less frequent and homeopathic remedies are relatively tasteless. The remedy that best fits the signs in patients is used.

Bi Yan Pian (nose inflammation tablet): This herbal formula is appropriate for upper respiratory infections in which sneezing and nasal discharge (especially mucopurulent) predominate.

Gan Mao Ling: This herbal formula is appropriate for patients in which pharyngeal and upper tracheal signs predominate.[17,22,23]

Colostrum provides proteoglycans used during the immune response to viruses and bacteria. Levels provided by the normal diet may not be sufficient during times of increased consumption due to viral and/or bacterial infections. Colostrum is also therapeutic for oral and GI irritation and ulceration.

Cod liver oil can be applied topically to eyes in the case of conjunctivitis and corneal ulceration. This treatment helps soothe the tissues of the eye and promotes healing of corneal ulcers. Oral administration is helpful as an antioxidant and for immune support.[17,30] However, because of its vitamin A content, dosing must be carefully calculated in pediatric patients.

For marshmallow root, a slurry made from the powdered form or diluted tincture can be used for patients with oral ulceration. It is soothing and protective for oral and GI irritation or ulceration.

Pill curing can be used to treat nausea secondary to postnasal drip ingestion.

Acupuncture is helpful for relieving pain, maintaining appetite, clearing mucus, and immune support.

Dermatologic Disease

Skin disease is generally a sign of underlying chronic disease. From a holistic perspective, skin disorders are the first level of disease. The severity of disease progresses from the distal and ventral skin moving upwards toward the head. If progression continues, physiologic and later pathologic changes move to internal organs. Patients that present with signs manifesting only in the skin have the highest likelihood of a curative response.

Otitis externa

Excessive earwax production and inflammation is generally associated with chronic disease. A thorough history and physical examination should be performed to identify any additional sign of disease. Treatments that support healthy immune functioning are generally indicated in cases that involve chronic or recurrent inflammation. An otoscopic examination to assess the competency of the tympanic membrane should precede any topical treatments.

Topicals and nutritional supplements

Almond oil is useful in cases of excessive earwax and mild otitis externa.[4,17] It dissolves wax and soothes irritated tissues.[4,17,30] In addition, it can be used to treat recurrent cases of ear mites or in cases when clients prefer a nonchemical method of treatment. Almond oil will suffocate mites and eggs. The treatment should be once to twice daily for 3 weeks to account for the mite life cycle. The author generally begins with more frequent treatment when abundant wax and inflammation are present and reduce to daily once the signs are improving. When continuous treatment is not possible because of patient compliance, treatment for 2 weeks followed by a 1-week break and treatment for an additional week is often sufficient.

Oral probiotics may be helpful in cases with bacterial or yeast overgrowth. Topically powdered probiotics can be applied in the ear once daily at bedtime. This is often extremely helpful for cases of chronic *Malassezia* otitis.

There are many herbal ear washes available on the market. These ear washes often contain herbals that reduce inflammation and have antimicrobial effects. They can be useful to reduce or eliminate the necessity for medicated ointments.

Demodicosis

Demodex is a normal commensal mite of dogs normally present is small numbers.[31,32] *Demodex* mites live in facial hair follicles, particularly around the periocular area. Demodicosis is categorized as either localized or generalized. Localized *Demodex* in puppies does not show a familial pattern of occurrence. More than 90% of prepubertal dogs with localized demodicosis resolve spontaneously in 3 to 8 weeks. This resolution is thought to occur as the puppy becomes more immunocompetent with age. Generalized *Demodex* is a familial disease problem. Most cases of generalized demodicosis begin as local lesions. Pruritus, inflammation, and secondary bacterial overgrowths often accompany cases of generalized demodicosis.

Treatment of Demodicosis

Cases of demodicosis are treated on an individual basis. Most patients will benefit from immune-enhancing herbal formulas matched to their specific pattern of disease. Herbals with antiinflammatory effects in the skin and that reduce pruritus are helpful. These herbals, in addition to calming formulas, can help to reduce self-trauma and improve the emotional status of patients.

Topicals and nutritional supplements

Probiotics enhance systemic immunity and are helpful in supporting a normal floral ecology.[33,34]

Green tea/black tea can be used topically for its antimicrobial, antiinflammatory, and antipruritic effects.[17]

Calendula is a nonalcoholic herbal or homeopathic spray (solution) that can be used topically for antiinflammatory, antimicrobial, and antipruritic effects.[2,4,17]

Flea allergy dermatitis

Healthy individuals do not show signs of flea allergy dermatitis. They do not require chemical flea treatments to remain free from evidence of fleas. In severe infestations with significant signs, chemical flea treatments with rapid onset may be required. Ongoing control can be easily achieved for most individuals without the use of spot-on or oral antiflea chemicals. The routine use of non-chemical flea control reserves the use of chemicals for patients with significant clinical signs attributable to flea sensitivity. Reducing the widespread use of flea control chemicals may help to preserve their efficacy through reduced resistance. In addition, it removes exposure of patients, other animals, clients, and children in the household to these chemicals.

Natural Flea Control

Boric acid (salt) is a detergent powder that removes the wax coating on the flea causing it to die from desiccation. Toxicologic evaluation results show it to be less toxic than table salt. It is applied to the environment (not the patients). It is guaranteed effective for 1 year.

B vitamin supplementation seems to reduce the number of fleas attracted to patients. Experimental trials of various B vitamin supplements have shown inconsistent results as a repellent. There is often more than a 3-week delay in improvement of flea numbers, which may indicate changes other than a direct repellent effect (ie, reduced skin inflammation) may be the cause of improvements. B vitamins have antioxidant and immune-supportive actions,[30] which may be beneficial in improving the signs of flea allergy dermatitis. There are several products for oral supplementation including B vitamins along with herbs known to have antipruritic and calming effects.

Neem has an insect repellent effect and is an antiinflammatory as well as an antimicrobial.[2] There are shampoos and sprays available containing neem, often in conjunction with other herbs (eg, citronella, eucalyptus) with insect-repelling effects.

Balanced diets low in carbohydrates and without preservatives or added chemicals often greatly reduce evidence of fleas.

RESOURCES FOR VETERINARIANS

Many herbal and nutraceutical companies provide support for veterinarians, assisting with proper formula selection, dosing, drug interactions, and contraindications. The following is a partial list of companies commonly used by the author as a resource for practitioners:

Dr Xie's Jing-tang Herbal Inc: www.tcvmherbal.com; telephone: 800-891-1986; address: 9700 West Highway 318, Reddick, FL 32686

Golden Flower Chinese Herbs: www.gfcherbs.com; telephone: 800-729-8509; address: 2724 Vassar Place NE, Albuquerque, NM 87107

Health Concerns: www.healthconcerns.com; telephone: 800-233-9355; address: 8001 Capwell Drive, Oakland, CA 94621

Kan Herb Company: www.kanherb.com; telephone: 800-543-5233; address: 380 Encinal Street Suite 100, Santa Cruz, CA 95060

Thorne Research: www.veterinary.thorne.com; telephone: 800-228-1966; address: PO Box 25, Dover, ID 83825

REFERENCES

1. McKean E. The New Oxford American Dictionary. 2nd Edition. New York: Oxford University Press; 2005. p. 806.
2. Gruenwald J, Brendler T, Jaenicke C, et al. PDR for herbal medicines. 4th edition. Montvale (NJ): Thompson Healthcare Inc; 2007. p. 194–5, 559–61, 569–70, 755–6.
3. Bensky D, Gamble A. Chinese herbal medicine materia medica revised edition. Seattle (WA): Eastland Press, Inc; 1993. p. 49–50.
4. Picairn R, Hubble Pitcairn S. Dr Pitcairn's complete guide to natural health for dogs & cats. 3rd edition. Emmaus (PA): Rodale; 2005. p. 264–5, 344.
5. Hamilton D. Homeopathic care for cats and dogs – small doses for small animals. Berkeley (CA): North Atlantic Books; 1999. p. 6–7, 14.
6. Vithoulkas G. The science of homeopathy. New York: Grove Press; 1980. p. 80, 104.
7. Magne M. Selected topics in pediatric gastroenterology. Vet Clin North Am Small Anim Pract 2006;36:533–48.
8. Hoskin JD, Dimski D. The digestive system. In: Hoskins JD, editor. Veterinary pediatrics. 2nd edition. Philadelphia: WB Saunders; 1990. p. 133–87.
9. Camichael LE, Schlafer DH, Hashimoto A. Minute virus of canines (MVC, canine parvovirus type-1): pathogenicity for pups and seroprevalence estimate. J Vet Diagn Invest 1994;6(2):165–74.
10. Rothrock K. 2012 Nov 30. Minute virus infection. Associate database. VIN.com. Available at: http://www.vin.com/Members/Associate/Associate.plx?DiseaseId=5549. Accessed August 3, 2013.
11. Sherding R. Diseases of the intestines. In: Birchard S, Sherding R, editors. Saunders manual of small animal practice. Philadelphia: WB Saunders Co; 1994. p. 687–714.
12. Chorazy ML, Richardson DJ. A survey of environmental contamination with ascarid ova, Wallingford, Connecticut. Vector Borne Zoonotic Dis 2005;5(1): 33–9.
13. Reinemeyer CR. Canine gastrointestinal parasites. In: Bonagura JD, editor. Kirk's current veterinary therapy. 12th edition. Philadelphia: WB Saunders Co; 1995. p. 711–6.
14. Roddie G, Stafford P, Holland C, et al. Contamination of dog hair with eggs of Toxocara canis. Vet Parasitol 2008;152(1–2):85–93. http://dx.doi.org/10.1016/j.vetpar.2007.12.008.
15. Becker AC, Rohen M, Epe C, et al. Prevalence of endoparasites in stray and fostered dogs and cats in Northern Germany. Parasitol Res 2012;111(2):849–57.
16. Leib MS, Zajac AM. Giardia: diagnosis and treatment. In: Bonagura JD, editor. Kirk's current veterinary therapy. 12th edition. Philadelphia: WB Saunders Co; 1995. p. 716–20.
17. Schwartz C. Four paws five directions: a guide to Chinese medicine for cats & dogs. Berkeley (CA): Ten Speed Press; 1996. p. 167, 171, 180, 189, 220, 322–3, 328.
18. Hammett T. Non-timber forest product. Factsheet number 17. 2001 Jan. Special Forest Products Program at Virginia Tech in collaboration with: USDA Forest Service, Southern Research Station. FREC.VT.edu. Available at: http://www.sfp.forprod.vt.edu/factsheets/clm.pdf. Accessed August 3, 2013.

19. Deters A, Zippel J, Hellenbrand N, et al. Aqueous extracts and polysaccharides from marshmallow roots (Althea officinalis L.): cellular internalization and stimulation of cell physiology of human epithelial cells in vitro. J Ethnopharmacol 2010; 127(1):62–9. http://dx.doi.org/10.1016/j.jep.2009.09.050.

20. Watt K, Christofi N, Young R. The detection of antibacterial actions of whole herb tinctures using luminescent Escherichia coli. Phytother Res 2007;21(12):1193–9.

21. Lauk L, Lo Bue AM, Milazzo I, et al. Antibacterial activity of medicinal plant extracts against periodontopathic bacteria. Phytother Res 2003;17(6): 599–604.

22. Scott J, Monda L, Heuertz J. Clinical guide to commonly used Chinese herbal formulas. 5th edition. Placitas (NM): Herbal Medicine Press; 2011. p. 16, 24, 33.

23. Fratkin J. Chinese herbal patent formulas a practical guide. 10th edition. Boulder (CO): Shya Publications; 1997. p. 52–3, 64, 70, 162.

24. Maciocia G. The practice of Chinese medicine: the treatment of diseases with acupuncture and Chinese herbs. Edinburgh (United Kingdom): Churchill Livingstone; 1998. p. 74–5, 168–9, 391, 404, 439, 789–90.

25. Playford RJ, Floyd DN, Macdonald CE, et al. Bovine colostrum is a health food supplement which prevents NSAID induced gut damage. Gut 1999;44(5):653–8.

26. Xu RJ. Development of the newborn GI tract and its relation to colostrum/milk intake: a review. Reprod Fertil Dev 1996;8(1):35–48.

27. Struff WG, Sprotte G. Bovine colostrum as a biologic in clinical medicine: a review–part II: clinical studies. Int J Clin Pharmacol Ther 2008;46(5):211–25.

28. Johnson LR. 2012. Update on respiratory pathogens. Western Veterinary Conference. VIN.com. Available at: http://www.vin.com/doc/?id=5604005. Accessed August 3, 2013.

29. Taboada J, Turnwald GH. The respiratory system. In: Hoskins JD, editor. Veterinary pediatrics. 2nd edition. Philadelphia: WB Saunders; 1990. p. 71–93.

30. Hendler SS, Rorvik D, editors. PDR for nutritional supplements. 2nd edition. Montvale (NJ): Physicians' Desk Reference Inc; 2008. p. 98–100, 634–54.

31. Nagle T. Topics in pediatric dermatology. Vet Clin North Am Small Anim Pract 2006;36:557–72.

32. Foil C. The skin. In: Hoskins JD, editor. Veterinary pediatrics. 2nd edition. Philadelphia: WB Saunders; 1990. p. 227–82.

33. Bowe WP, Patel NB, Logan AC. Acne vulgaris, probiotics and the gut-brain-skin axis: from anecdote to translational medicine. Benef Microbes 2013 July 25;1–15.

34. Jung BG, Cho SJ, Koh HB, et al. Fermented Maesil (Prunus mume) with probiotics inhibits development of atopic dermatitis-like skin lesions in NC/Nga mice. Vet Dermatol 2010;21(2):184–91. http://dx.doi.org/10.1111/j.1365-3164.2009.00796.x.

Index

Note: Page numbers of article titles are in **boldface** type.

A

Aciduria
    L-2 hydroxyglutaric
        in puppies, 280–281
Adenovirus
    in puppies
        2013 update on, 245
Anatomic anomalies
    in juvenile dogs, 314–318
Ankyloglossia
    in dogs, 305
Anticonvulsant(s)
    in seizure disorder management in puppies and kittens, 290–296
        benzodiazepines, 294
        bromide, 292
        felbamate, 293–294
        gabapentin, 293
        levetiracetam, 292
        monitoring of, 295–296
        phenobarbital, 291–292
        pregabalin, 293
        zonisamide, 292–293

B

Benign prostatic hypertrophy (BPH)
    decreased risk of
        pediatric gonadectomy and, 224
Benzodiazepines
    in seizure disorder management in puppies and kittens, 294
Bitch(es)
    pregnant and lactating
        nutrition for, 265–267
Bordetella spp.
    in kittens
        vaccine for
            2013 update on, 253
    in puppies
        vaccine for
            2013 update on, 247
Bordetellosis
    in cats, 335–336

Vet Clin Small Anim 44 (2014) 367–378
http://dx.doi.org/10.1016/S0195-5616(14)00020-5
0195-5616/14/$ – see front matter © 2014 Elsevier Inc. All rights reserved.

Moving?

Make sure your subscription moves with you!

To notify us of your new address, find your **Clinics Account Number** (located on your mailing label above your name), and contact customer service at:

Email: **journalscustomerservice-usa@elsevier.com**

800-654-2452 (subscribers in the U.S. & Canada)
314-447-8871 (subscribers outside of the U.S. & Canada)

Fax number: **314-447-8029**

Elsevier Health Sciences Division
Subscription Customer Service
3251 Riverport Lane
Maryland Heights, MO 63043

*To ensure uninterrupted delivery of your subscription, please notify us at least 4 weeks in advance of move.

Printed and bound by CPI Group (UK) Ltd, Croydon, CR0 4YY

03/10/2024

01040488-0015